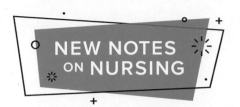

NEW NOTES
ON NURSING

HOW TO BE A SUCCESSFUL NURSING STUDENT

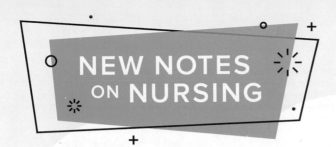

NEW NOTES ON NURSING

HOW TO BE A SUCCESSFUL NURSING STUDENT

EDITOR

Natalie Elliott, BSc (Hons) Adult Nursing

SERIES EDITOR

Teresa Chinn, MBE, RN, QN

CONSULTING EDITOR

June Girvin

ELSEVIER

ISBN: 978-0-323-88179-1

Content Strategist: Robert Edwards
Content Project Manager: Shivani Pal
Design: Renee Duenow

Printed in India

Last digit is the print number: 9   8   7   6   5   4   3   2   1

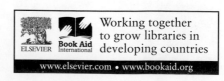

CONTRIBUTORS

Katie Anderson, BA Nursing (Child)

Helen Davis, BSc Nursing, RNCB, PGCert

Chelsea Fawcett, BSc Mental Health Nursing

Emma Hall, Student Nurse, CYPStNN Deputy Lead

Simon James, BSc Adult Nursing

Paul Jebb, MA, BSc (Hons), DipHE

Rebecca Lowe, MSc Adult Nursing

Heather Louise Massie, BSc Adult Nursing

Kelvin McMillan, BSc Nursing

Eula Eudolah Miller, EdD, MSc Research, RGN, RMN, DipHE Com. Health, Dip. Counselling, PGCE, RNT, MHFA Instructor, MBACP, SFHEA

Calvin Moorley, BA (Hons), PhD, RN

Gayatri Nambiar-Greenwood, BSc (Hons), MA (Hons), PhD, RGN

Joy O'Gorman, BSc (Hons) Adult Nursing

Hetal Patel, FHEA

Christie Roberts, BSc, RN

Joshua Sharman, BSc (Hons) Adult Nursing MSc Public Health

Stuart Tuckwood, Bachelor of Nursing (Hons), MSc Public Health

Sally Wilson, RNLD, MSc, RCN

Elisha Woolf, BSc Adult Nursing

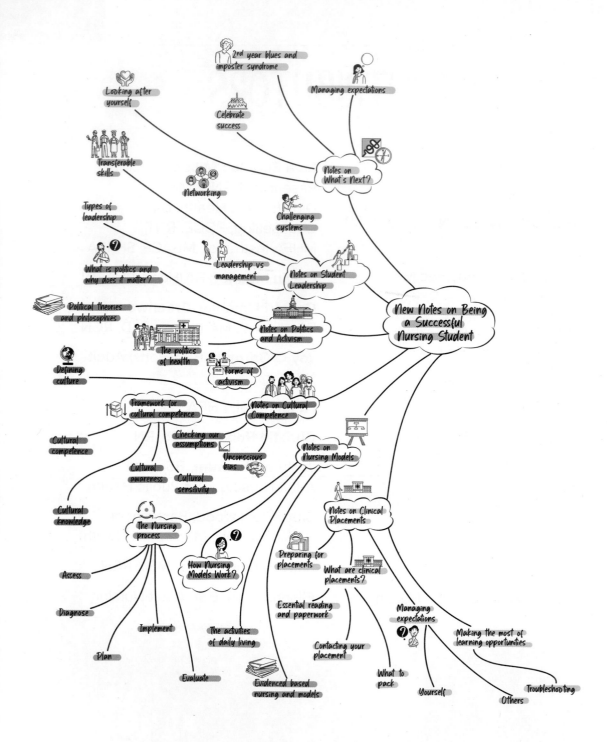

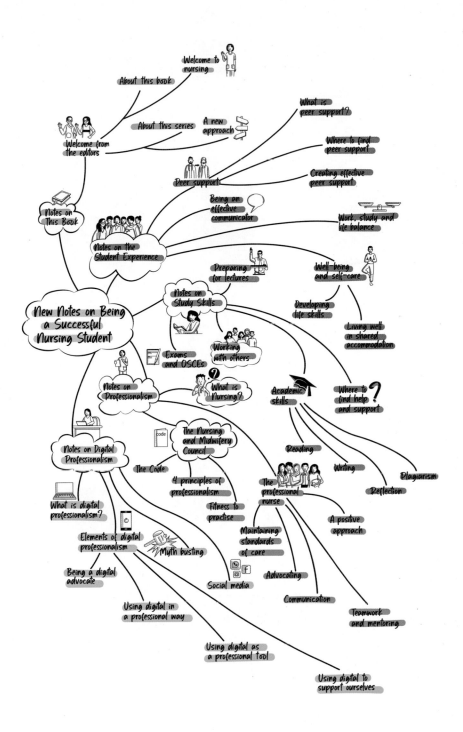

New Notes on Being a Successful Nursing Student

Welcome to nursing
About this book
Welcome from the editors
About this series
A new approach
Notes on This Book

What is peer support?
Where to find peer support
Creating effective peer support
Peer support

Notes on the Student Experience
Being an effective communicator
Work, study and life balance
Well-being and self-care
Developing life skills
Living well in shared accommodation

Preparing for lectures
Notes on Study Skills
Working with others
Exams and OSCEs

Academic skills
Where to find help and support

What is Nursing?
Notes on Professionalism

The Nursing and Midwifery Council
Reading
The professional nurse
Writing
Plagiarism
Reflection
A positive approach

Notes on Digital Professionalism
The Code
4 principles of professionalism
Fitness to practise
Maintaining standards of care
Advocating
Communication
Teamwork and mentoring

What is digital professionalism?
Elements of digital professionalism
Myth busting
Being a digital advocate
Social media
Using digital in a professional way
Using digital as a professional tool
Using digital to support ourselves

CONTENTS

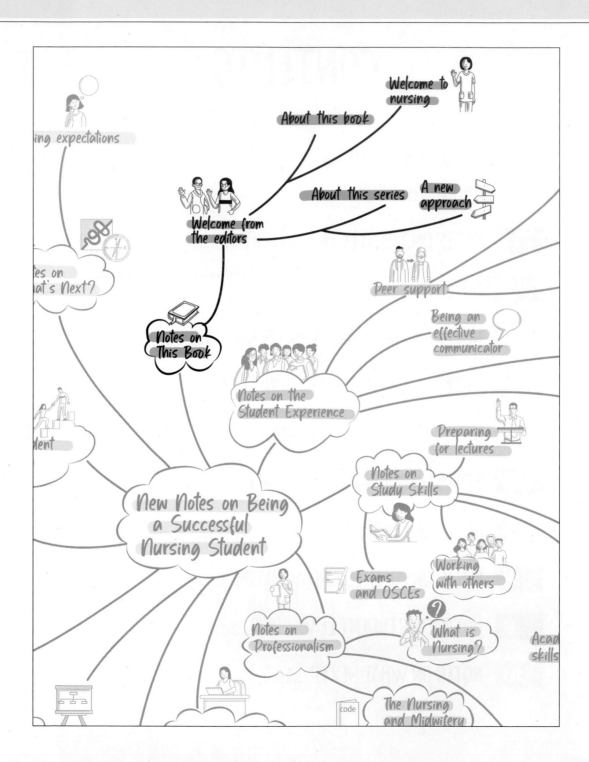

ABOUT THIS SERIES

Teresa Chinn (She/Her) ■ **June Girvin (She/Her)**

DEAR NURSING STUDENT

We are pleased that you have chosen this book from the other nursing books on the shelf! You may have noticed that it appears different from other books in the nursing section and there's a very good reason for that – it is different! This is the first in a series of books aimed at supporting you as a nursing student. The series combines a nursing book and a digital perspective, including the use of social media, that we hope will create a user-friendly and engaging approach to some of the fundamental topics and challenges in nursing.

The title for the series *New Notes on Nursing* is respectfully and humbly borrowed from Florence Nightingale's own writing. Her *Notes on Nursing* (1860), outlined a vision for health and wellness that encompassed social, political, economic, and environmental determinants as well as public health and illness prevention – the bigger picture within which good nursing care must be grounded. We recognise that for many new nursing students, some of the concepts that inform nursing can be challenging and complex, and may not always appear immediately relevant. The *New Notes...* series seeks to address that. We have tried hard to present content in a friendly style, conversational as far as possible, and incorporating social media so that interacting with this book is not a solitary activity but one that can be shared with others who are using the same book and finding out about the same things – whether they are in your cohort or somewhere else in the UK.

We are trying new design approaches using colourful and engaging content that is aimed at helping you identify the information you need quickly and easily. We understand that sometimes you don't want (or need) to read a dense textbook from start to finish to pull out the most helpful information for your situation, but rather easily identify the bits that are relevant for you at a point in time. We think our colour-coding and infographics throughout the books will help you do just that. We have also included all sorts of helpful 'sidenotes'; again taking inspiration from Florence Nightingale's writing:

THE CODE SAYS

These show the part of the code that the text is relevant to, helping you to embed the code into every area of your practice and thinking.

TWEET

'These are tweets from Registered Nurses and nursing students that share snippets of wisdom and perspective'

We have asked many people to contribute to the New Notes on Nursing books *and we have included some long quotes from these people; these have been especially written for this series.*

CASE STUDY

Case studies, both real and imagined, are a great way to put learning into context so you will find plenty of them in this series.

Your notes are just as important as ours and you will find lots of space in *New Notes on Nursing* for your own notes.

_____

_____

_____

_____

_____

_____

_____

_____

We have created the books with neurodiversity in mind and have tried to ensure that there is a feeling of space and lightness to the book.

In addition to all of this, we really want to engage and support you on your nursing student journey, so we have created some social media resources for you to tap into. Please search #NewNotesOnNursing and #SuccessfulStN on Twitter to find out more.

The team of Editors and Authors that we have asked to contribute to *New Notes on Nursing* are all practising health and care professionals, ranging in experience from nursing students and newly qualified Registered Nurses to registered professionals working in clinical and education settings with a wealth of experience. They all wanted to help you. By inviting a variety of voices to create these books, we are sharing many perspectives with you. We hope it helps you to develop well-rounded views on which to start your nursing career.

You are the latest generation of nursing students, and we are so pleased and honoured to be, in some small way, supporting you to flourish. We really hope you enjoy this book (yes, enjoy!) and that, at the end of your student journey, it contains lots of notes scribbled by you, the pages are dog-eared, and the cover well-worn – a new generation of nursing texts for a new generation of Registered Nurses.

Today's nursing is socially complex, politically enmeshed, and at times finding its way through conflict and controversy to give the best holistic, person-centred care. We think it's the best career in the world.

Best wishes

June and Teresa

The series is edited by:

'I've been a Registered Nurse since 1996 and have made my career in the social care sector. In 2012 set up the nursing Twitter community @WeNurses to help bring together nurses from diverse spheres of practice. I was awarded an MBE for services to nursing in 2014 and in 2018, I was named one of the 70 most influential nurses from 1948 to 2018 by the Royal College of Nursing. I communicate in many different ways in the UK and Europe, particularly on the use of social media in Nursing. I was made a Queens Nurse in 2022'.

Teresa Chinn MBE QN @WeNurses

'I qualified as a Registered Nurse in 1976 and have spent a (very) long career in clinical and academic practice. I retired in 2017 and now work independently in roles committed to supporting individual nurses and nursing as a profession – writing, commentating, coaching, reviewing, etc. I was delighted to be asked to support the development of this new series of books and to work with the team of writers/editors and Elsevier'.

June Girvin @ProfJuneG

Reflection boxes appear at the end of each chapter to enable and encourage post chapter reflection.

_____

_____

_____

_____

_____

_____

_____

_____

_____

_____

_____

_____

_____

_____

_____

_____

REFERENCES

Nightingale, Florence. 1860. Notes on nursing: what it is, and what it is not. London: Harrison. Harvard (18th ed.).

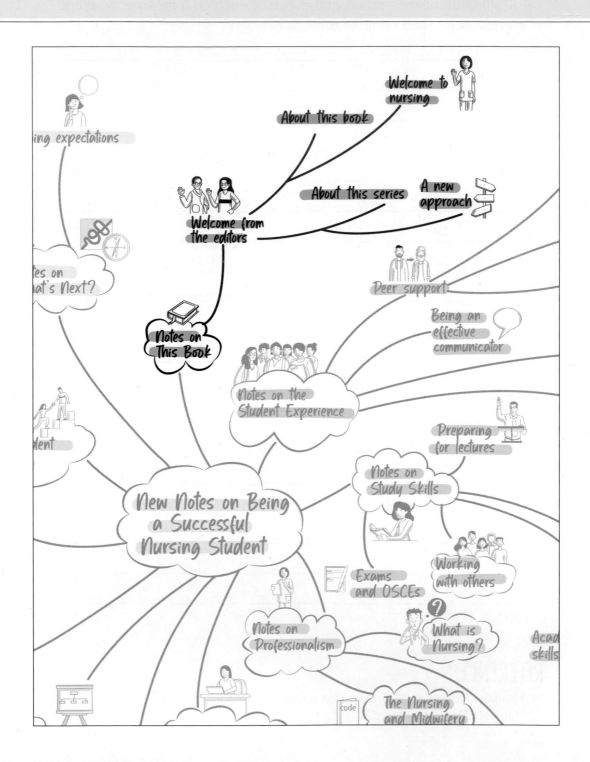

ABOUT THIS BOOK

Natalie Elliott (She/Her)

DEAR NURSING STUDENT

Hello and welcome to this book, *How to be a Successful Nursing Student*, and welcome to the world of nursing! The next few years are going to push you completely out of your comfort zone. There will be times you question your sanity, and there will be times when you question why you didn't become a Registered Nurse sooner.

I won't lie, a nursing degree is not an easy undertaking. It's emotionally, physically, and socially challenging, but despite the demands, becoming a Registered Nurse is 100% worth it. You will be privileged to meet and learn from some truly remarkable people. You will be part of people's journeys at the most challenging points of their lives, and you will witness some of the most beautiful moments which will stay with you for a lifetime. You will learn skills that you probably didn't realise were important, and through reflection, you will develop as a person and come out the other side stronger.

As with many nursing books, the authors for each chapter of this book are highly experienced in their respective areas but what makes this book unique is that most of the chapters are written in collaboration with a nursing student (or newly Registered Nurse who has recently gone through the journey of being a nursing student). The information presented to you will be relevant and will emphasise key points that you need to know, making it an essential book for pre-registration nursing students.

This book is unlike any of the books on your bookshelf. It has been designed to be inclusive and interactive. Throughout the book, you will be encouraged to pause and reflect to gain a deeper understanding of the concepts covered. To help with this, there will be a series of case studies embedded throughout each chapter, which will bridge the gap between theory and reality. You will also see lots of tweets throughout the chapters from nursing students, lecturers, Registered Nurses, and many more people – we wanted this book to be practical and full of valuable hints and tips to help support you. The structure of the book is designed to guide you through the first year of the nursing course, starting with how to make the most of your time at university and why it's important to seize opportunities, ending with looking forward to the next part of your course – it's not as scary as you might think.

Some of you may have experience of health and social care, but for some of you, this is a completely new concept. I was new to the world of nursing when I started my degree, and I was completely unaware of what Registered Nurses do. That doesn't mean that my previous experiences and skills weren't transferable. There were also many people who had various experiences – some working in care homes, and some working for the NHS. The thing I loved about this is that we were all able to share our knowledge and experiences.

There may be stereotypes associated with nursing, none of which are true, but there is no bigger privilege than being able to play a small part in a person's life when they are at their most vulnerable. Whether it's comforting the parents of child who is seriously ill or helping an older person with their daily living tasks, or empowering a person with learning disabilities to become more independent or supporting a person with their mental health at a challenging time in their life. We end up giving a little part of ourselves to each person and that is what makes nursing so special.

WHAT IS NURSING?

Registered Nurses must have a strong moral compass to ensure that ethical judgements are made and that care always remains focused on the person, making them the first and foremost priority. We do this through the use of clinical judgement to provide holistic care to people which is founded on the best available research. It's about empowering people to achieve the best quality of life regardless of their disease or disability.

Registered Nurses work autonomously and collaboratively with others to ensure that people, regardless of their age, culture, or background, receive the best possible care. Nursing isn't only about caring for people who are ill but also about the promotion of health and prevention of illness through the education of others.

In the UK, nursing students need to complete 4,600 hours of education which is split between theory and practice – it might seem like a lot, but it's broken down into manageable chunks over the whole of your programme. Of course, nursing is so vast and varied that nursing educational programmes can only provide the foundations of your learning; there is a lot of work and research you need to do on your own to become the best Registered Nurse you possibly can be.

When you applied for university, you will have chosen a specialism (also known as fields or branches) to focus on for the entirety of your degree. There are four specialisms – adult nursing, children's nursing, mental health nursing, and learning disability nursing. It is always good to understand what the other fields of practice do besides your own.

Adult nursing

This field of nursing works mainly with people over the age of 18 and is a general specialism. Registered Nurses try to understand and consider a patient's emotional and social problems as well as their medical condition. Adult Registered Nurses come across patients with a wide range of physical illnesses and injuries. Within a hospital setting, you may find that the wards are primarily broken down by each of the body systems (e.g. cardiology, renal, neurology, etc.). Adult Registered Nurses, however, are not just confined to hospital settings; they can also work in community (primary and third-sector) settings such as people's homes, health centres, nursing homes, reablement centres, and clinics, to name but a few!

Children's and young persons (CYP) nursing

CYP (or paediatric as it is sometimes called) Registered Nurses work with children and young people up to 19 years old and can work in a variety of settings, from specialist baby care units to adolescent units. It is not as simple as miniaturising adult nursing concepts as children react to illness in a very different way. Children often develop symptoms more extremely and more suddenly than adults, so CYP Registered Nurses must learn to be very careful observers and be able to recognise even the smallest of change in behaviour. CYP Registered Nurses also support, advise, and educate parents and carers.

Learning disability nursing

This field of nursing helps people from across the whole life span with learning disabilities to live independent and fulfilling lives. They help improve a person's physical and mental health whilst helping to reduce the barriers to the person living an independent life. They may work with people in supported accommodation, or with those who need more intensive support – for instance, in hospitals or in specialist secure units for offenders with learning disabilities.

Mental health nursing

Mental health problems can affect people of all ages and backgrounds. Patients' problems may be related to drug or alcohol use, childhood experiences, or particularly stressful situations. Mental Heath Registered Nurses help people control their mental health problems, cope better with life, and, where possible, recover. Mental Health Registered Nurses plan and deliver care for people in a variety of settings – such as at home or in specialist hospital services.

NURSING: PROFESSION OR VOCATION

Understanding the role of the Registered Nurse is one thing but understanding what made us a profession is just as important. How has modern nursing developed throughout the years, and how do we ensure that high standards of nursing care are delivered?

Florence Nightingale was undoubtedly the matriarch of the nursing profession in the late 1800s. However, Ethel Gordon Fenwick, who also was a nurse around at this time, equally had a profound impact on the nursing profession we know today. Fenwick, a former matron of St Bartholomew's Hospital in London, spent 30 years campaigning for the mandatory registration of nurses. She was concerned about varying training standards of nursing care and passionately believed that nurses should be brought together under one profession. She considered it to be important for nurses to have a standardised training programme and a single-entry route into nursing career. Through her advocacy, Ms Fenwick's efforts led to the Nurses Registration Act 1919.

Fast forward to 2001, when we see the inception of the Nursing and Midwifery Council (NMC) – the professional regulators of modern nursing. The main role of the NMC is to regulate nurses and midwives in the UK, and nursing associates in England, ensuring high-quality care is delivered consistently to the public. They also hold a register (remember Ethel Gordon Fenwick's activism?) of all the professionals who are eligible to practice. Lastly, they investigate concerns about Registered Nurses, Midwives, and Nursing Associates safeguarding the public.

The NMC also set standards, guidance, and requirements for nursing and midwifery education across the UK. These standards help to shape the content and design of nursing programmes and state what a Registered Nurse, Midwife or Nursing Associate needs to know and be able to do in order to deliver high-quality, person-centred care.

When students successfully complete their programme, their educational institution will let the NMC know that they have met the education and practice standards and are of good health and good character. You will then be considered fit to practise and will be eligible to apply to join the register – it might seem like forever away, but it'll be here before you know it!

There is, of course, much more to the history of nursing and if you have time, you should consider researching it more. It helps us understand where we are now.

DEFINING SUCCESS

Success is a dynamic notion, and what one person defines as being successful may be different to what another person wants their journey to look like. Equally, what you deem to be success may be different from your university/practice assessor/practice supervisor. Everyone's concept of success will likely be fluid with constant change over time.

> *'Success is going from failure to failure without losing enthusiasm'.*
>
> **– Winston Churchill**

> *'It is hard work, perseverance, learning, studying, sacrifice and most of all, love of what you are doing or learning to do'*
>
> **– Pele, Brazilian former professional footballer**

Success is unique to the individual and, therefore, success will be unique to you because we all have a different mix of talents and goals. Therefore, it is important that you start to think about what being 'a Successful Nursing Student' means to you.

Here are what some other people consider to be 'successful'

I have worked in healthcare in various roles for 12 years coupled with a few travelling trips to volunteer for disaster relief programs. And throughout this time, humanity always hits me right in the feels, specifically the children having to go through life in such tragic and unfair situation. I chose Children's nursing, because children are the future, they are our present, they deserve nothing but our best to either make them more comfortable in their conditions, they deserve us to fight and advocate for their needs,

and they deserve the best evidenced based practice we can give whilst innovating new ways to treat and care for them.

Success is the tide of many. It is a collaborative, passionate, professional, trailblazing group of individuals globally acting as a tide to promote the best patient outcomes; the best outcomes for humanity. And to quote Wen Kang, Not JFK! "A rising tide lifts all boats!!" That is what success means to me.

To be authentic, to be true, to really apply yourself, listen to others, listen to yourself, know when to take a break and when to go full throttle. To always remember why you are doing what you are doing.

 TIP

Every day, start with saying 'I can'. Finish the day by saying 'I did'. Drink lots of water. Go outside on your breaks from studying or being on the wards. Eat well. Get a good pen.

Sam Palmer, Children's Nursing, Year 2, London South Bank University, @Samchumba3

 I had always wanted to be a Registered Nurse from before leaving school but due to not getting the right grades, I had given up on the idea. After having my children, I took the route of working as a TA in a school, working mainly with SEND children and completed an education degree. After 15 years in education, I left to teach Yoga and mindfulness, and during that time I started teaching Yoga in my local hospital in a female acute ward. This made me want to finally embark on my Registered Nurse training in Mental

Continued

health nursing. I applied in March 2018 and starting my training in September 2018.

Success can mean different things according to whether it applies to academic work or practice. Academic work is a challenge for me, so anything above a pass is success, and as I have gone through the years, my academic work has improved, which again in success. In practice, success could mean knowing I have done my best that day. So, in mental health nursing, it could mean having a simple conversation with a service user/patient, making someone a cup of tea, getting a report written to support a tribunal, supporting my colleagues. Success to me, in a nutshell, is making a difference to the team and service users/ patients, and if I didn't reflect on where I can improve and learn.

Access all the support uni can offer you, e.g., academic support, wellbeing support, your personal academic tutor. Drop in for assignment/practice support. Talk to someone if you are struggling as chances are everyone has felt like you. Your wellbeing is important so look after yourself. There is never a 'silly question' - chances are other people are thinking the same thing.

TIP

Do use the read aloud function in word once you have completed an assignment - it is great.

Do speak up if in practice you are not getting support or have not been allocated a practice assessor etc.

Do plan on what you want to achieve in placement.

Do follow @westudentnurses on Twitter for great content, chat, and revision sessions, and a way of connecting with others.

Do join a union.

Don't feel alone, seek help and support because it can be hard fitting everything in. Everyone feels like this, but DON'T neglect your health and wellbeing.

Nikhola Haley, Mental Health Nursing Student, Year 3, University of Huddersfield, Twitter handle:@nikkilouh

Before you dive into the next chapter, have a think about what a successful year would look like for you. Are there any goals you want to achieve? Any comfort zones you want to push out of? It might help to think about why you chose nursing as a career and why you selected your specific field of practice. Perhaps even write some notes in the space below:

_____

_____

_____

_____

_____

_____

_____

Come back to this page throughout your nursing student journey, as this will help you to assess how you are progressing. It's also a good idea to return to this page when times are difficult to remind you exactly why you want to become a Registered Nurse.

Finally, I want to wish you the best of luck for the year ahead. I'd love to follow your journey and see how you become a successful nursing student, so please do connect with me not on Twitter (@nursing_nat) and share your journey using #SuccessfulStN. I am really looking forward to hearing about and celebrating all of your successes.

Kindest regards,

Natalie

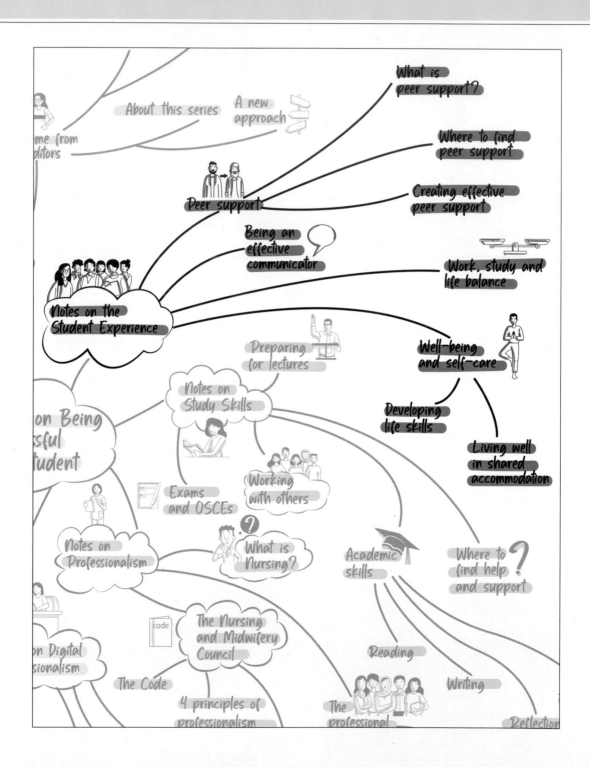

NOTES ON THE STUDENT EXPERIENCE

Katie Anderson (She/Her)

Kelvin McMillan (He/Him) ■ Helen Davis-Miles (She/Her)

INTRODUCTION

You have accepted your place on your chosen course and desired university and are hopefully excited to begin your nursing journey. Congratulations! As you now transition to higher education you are encouraged to immerse yourself in the full student experience. However, let's pause for a moment and consider what is meant by student experience.

Student experience within higher education encompasses all aspects of university life such as academic, social, political, cultural, and sporting interactions. This can be broken down further into key concepts such as teaching methods and quality, curriculum design, student facilities, student support, and course delivery, for example.

Unlike other courses, your nursing course will span the whole of the year. Therefore, you may not have a long summer break and instead may undertake placements. This is different to your peers studying alternative courses. The rationale for undertaking your course throughout the year is a condition by The Nursing and Midwifery Council (NMC) which requires you to undertake your course within the allocated time frame of your programme.

Your student experience of university is unique and will differ to that of other students as you will spend 50% in theory and 50% in practice. This will enable you to draw upon a range of learning environments and opportunities which will enhance your student experience.

Part of your student experience is getting to know your peers. It's a unique bond that you will form sharing your journey as well as reflecting upon experiences or situations you have been in. At times your course may be challenging and push you out of your comfort zone; therefore the support from peers will enable you to process and continue on your course as they too can relate to some of the thoughts and feelings you have experienced.

DEVELOPING PEER SUPPORT NETWORKS

Peer support in educational terms is supporting others by offering education, individual experiences, practical help, and feedback to benefit the learning needs of a group. Everyone's journey through life has been different; your motivation and drive to be where you are now will be different to others. Peer support can bring all these qualities together in one collective space, enhancing the learning environment, and as such enhance the student experience.

The qualities of peer support learning are highlighted below:

Educational experiences	The identification that educational needs and backgrounds are different but unique. The diversity of a peer group is celebrated, and acknowledgement of different learning requirements and personalities encourages a more inclusive environment.
Individual experiences	Life experience encourages empathy and alternative solutions to problems. Upbringing and environments can shape the way we think about problems and debates, promoting constructive conversation and feedback. Diversity of subject strengths and weaknesses should also be embraced, as it provides opportunities to teach each other.
Practical experiences	Acknowledging that individual peers learn differently and require different motivation to learn. It also acknowledges that individuals have different access requirements to technology and resources, as well as knowledge of accessing digital resources. Overcoming obstacles to help others' learning needs is critical to encouraging an inclusive and non-discriminatory environment.

Reflective skills	The ability to undertake formative assessment exercises such as group work, quizzes, or constructing presentations is done for the purpose of gaining feedback to benefit the whole group. A peer group reflects on feedback and discusses how development can be made effective.
Motivation and support	Having empathy for others and embracing that each peer has challenges in life. An effective peer group creates safe spaces for individuals to either be open and honest or allows the ability for individuals to reach out to others. If someone isn't as active within a peer group, it's an opportunity to reach out and generate solutions to promote equal opportunities for everyone.
Leadership qualities	A peer support group should not be overseen by one individual; it should allow overall transformation influenced by positive individual contributions. Constructive communication and ability to feedback are crucial to enhancing individual leadership qualities, which can result in valuable contributions being made to help the peer group.

Whilst peer support groups can lead to enhanced professional development, they can also lead to vital personal development, setting further foundations to develop your role as a future Registered Nurse. Other advantages include:

- Increased mental health support.
- More inclusive classroom.
- Higher achievement within the classroom.
- Higher achievement in assessments.
- Increased self-esteem.
- Enhanced self-advocacy skills.
- Improved positive behaviour.
- Increased attendance within lectures and placements.
- Development of positive and diverse relationships amongst peers.
- Enhancing problem-solving skills.

Once you become a Registered Nurse you will be required, under the NMC code of conduct, to continue this professional development.

NMC

THE CODE SAYS

22.3 Keep your knowledge and skills up to date, taking part in appropriate and regular learning and professional development activities that aim to maintain and develop your competence and improve your performance

How to create effective peer support groups?

As with any team, a successful peer support group requires time, patience, and planning. The more effort you put into these steps, the more successful your peer support group will be.

CASE STUDY

Peer Support Group named 'The ECGs'

The ECGs are a group of four third-year nursing students who have just started their first module of year 3. These individuals have been randomly selected by the module leader and are expected to work together throughout the nine-week module. They are expected to complete group work, a small presentation and pre-/post-lecture work.

Alice has appointed herself as a leader. Alice is a confident and knowledgeable individual who is not afraid to speak out and answer questions during lectures. The rest of the group consist of:

- Salma – an individual who academically is good but is not confident speaking her ideas.
- Tom – an individual who has underlying generalised anxiety and has often missed sessions due to his mental health.
- April – an individual who has dyslexia and has had family difficulties impacting her studies.

A small presentation is due in two weeks, and the ECGs have been assigned to present one ethical principle that impacts the Registered Nurses's role whilst developing an Advanced Care Plan (ACP) for a patient with a life-limiting condition. Alice provides a plan and allocates everyone with specific slides to complete. Alice tries to

CASE STUDY—cont'd

arrange regular meetings over Microsoft Teams but is struggling to get Tom and April to attend. Salma attends regularly but is very quiet during meetings, which frustrates Alice.

Two days before the presentation deadline, Alice checks to see if everyone has completed their slides. Salma completed her slides; however, Tom and April did not. Alice sends Tom and April an email expressing her frustration at Tom and April, accusing them both of not being team players. Alice receives replies from both Tom and April; Tom stated he has been in hospital due to self-harming, and April stated that her mother has been diagnosed with cancer and its terminal.

This case study is an example of individuals being allocated a peer group, and the dynamics simply not working. Alice as a leading voice should have considered getting to know April, Salma, and Tom before making concrete decisions.

Sometimes at university you will be offered an opportunity to choose your own peer groups, but sometimes like the ECGs, you will be allocated peer support groups on your behalf.

Think about what went wrong with the ECG's peer support group. What could have been done differently?

_____

_____

_____

_____

_____

_____

There are six steps for effective and successful peer support groups:

1. Break the ice – get to know each other.
2. Identify individual strengths and weaknesses.

3. Identify individual practical needs.
4. Create safe space(s).
5. Create the schedule.
6. Review the group dynamics.

Thinking about the ECGs, Alice did attempt to create safe spaces using Microsoft Teams; however, introductions and strengths were not recognised. Here are each of the steps broken down with ideas:

- Break the ice: create opportunities to get to know each other. For example, fun questions you can ask include, 'Who is your favourite cartoon character?' Or activities such as two truths and one lie or playing charades.
- Identify individual strengths and weaknesses: learn who has knowledge in key areas and practical strengths. For example, who is confident in anatomy and physiology? Who is not confident in anatomy and physiology?
- Identify individual practical needs: does everyone have equal opportunity to access resources? Who has specific travelling arrangements? Questions like these will help you plan how you regularly meet within your peer support groups.
- Create safe space(s): figure out what platform or environment will suit you all best. It might be a combination of environments such as having time in the library, as well as a social media space such as WhatsApp.
- Create a schedule: figure out a schedule that suits everyone's needs. Everyone has different responsibilities, so ensure everyone has opportunities to meet on a regular basis.
- Review: once the first five steps are in place, you can review how the peer support group is going. If you feel there are individual concerns, go back to step one and follow the process again to help that person.

Where can I find peer support networks?

Finding other peer support networks requires proactiveness and observation of opportunities that present themselves. Not only are peer support networks found within the foundations of the university walls or classroom, but they can also be found across a variety of learning/social platforms (Fig 1.1).

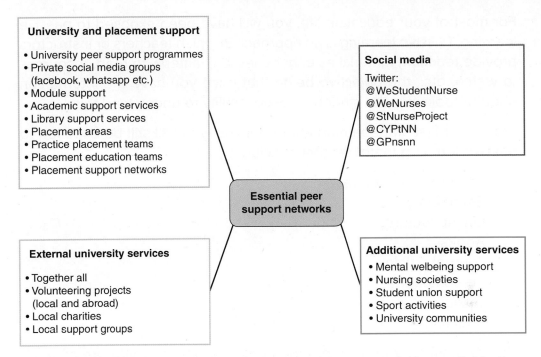

University and placement support

- University peer support programmes
- Private social media groups (facebook, whatsapp etc.)
- Module support
- Academic support services
- Library support services
- Placement areas
- Practice placement teams
- Placement education teams
- Placement support networks

Social media

Twitter:
@WeStudentNurse
@WeNurses
@StNurseProject
@CYPtNN
@GPnsnn

Essential peer support networks

External university services

- Together all
- Volunteering projects (local and abroad)
- Local charities
- Local support groups

Additional university services

- Mental welbeing support
- Nursing societies
- Student union support
- Sport activities
- University communities

Figure 1.1 Diagram showing important peer support networks available to nursing students whilst studying nursing at university.

'Don't be afraid to ask questions. Don't be afraid to ask for help when you need it. I do that every day. Asking for help is not a sign of weakness, it's a sign of strength. It shows you have courage to admit when you don't know something, and to learn something new.'

—The Obama White House, 2019

How to be an effective learner?

To make the most of your university experience, you need to develop independence in your learning. Nursing is a career of lifelong learning, but it is up to you to reach out for opportunities to better yourself.

'Learning is not the product of teaching. Learning is the product of the activity of learners.'

—Holt, 1984

For most of your education life, you will have been exposed to passive learning. Passive learning is an approach in which teachers or instructors provide teaching material as either a lesson, material to read, resources to watch, etc., the objective being that once you have the information about a topic, it is the student's responsibility to understand this.

When you first start learning about nursing, you will still be exposed to passive learning methods; these include:

- Face-to-face lectures
- Seminars
- Online lectures
- Books
- Journal articles
- Presentations
- Webinars
- Podcasts

However, when you walk into the nursing profession, you are committing yourself to lifelong learning.

NMC | THE CODE SAYS

6.2 Maintain the knowledge and skills you need for safe and effective practice (Nursing and Midwifery Council, 2018).

This means that you are going to need to generate learning opportunities to help you progress in your career and maintain the knowledge necessary to care for your patients. As nursing students, you will be expected to digest teaching and resources that are provided, but you are also expected to think about topics, challenge ideas, discuss the theory underpinning clinical practice, and analyse information. This requires an active learning approach.

The learning pyramid provides insight into the importance of engaging in active learning. You might have done active learning using group work during teaching sessions, or perhaps you might have presented in front of a group (Fig 1.2). These are all active learning opportunities; it

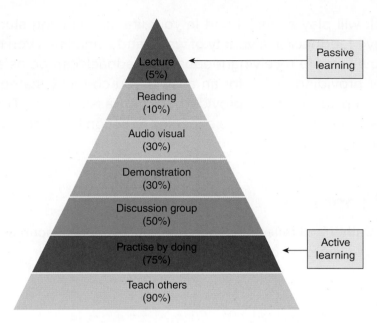

Figure 1.2   The Learning Pyramid, National Training Laboratory.

puts the emphasis on the students rather than it being teacher centred. As such, you will be expected to participate in active learning opportunities such as:

- Peer learning and teaching
- Presenting information
- Group work
- Case study activities
- Role play
- Simulation
- Group projects

To get the best out of your university experience, you must immerse yourself in what the university has to offer. This is what university life is all about; not only are you professionally developing yourself, but you are also personally developing yourself, so you are more career ready. It's like joining a gym for the first time; you often get provided with work-out plans designed to help you achieve your fitness goal. But over time, How will I know I am progressing in the right direction?

Feedback will play a crucial part in your life as a nursing student. You will receive feedback in a variety of ways, and sometimes you might not even know you are receiving feedback. Feedback can be as simple as a lecturer providing praise for an answer you correctly stated in a lecture, right up to feedback provided after an assessment. Throughout your nursing career, you will be expected to act on feedback to improve your clinical practice.

NMC

THE CODE SAYS

9.2 Gather and reflect on feedback from a variety of sources, using it to improve your practice and performance.

TWEET

@hannahlames1

There is a huge value on having your practice watched and receiving feedback for improvement in patient safety and experience as well as your own professional development.

Feedback can be provided through things such as:

- Teaching sessions
- Group work
- Peer group work
- Online quizzes
- Virtual learning environments
- Assessments
- Clinical practice supervisors and assessors
- Academic assessor/personal tutor meetings
- Skills and simulation
- Presentation feedback.
- Patient and family/service user feedback

MANAGING AND DEVELOPING A HEALTHY WORK/STUDY LIFE BALANCE

As you transition to university to begin your nursing career it's important to maintain a work/study life balance as well as your physical and mental wellbeing. Our physical and mental health can change from day to day, as some days can be more challenging than others. As a nursing student, you are in a unique position where your course includes theory and clinical modules. This means you will regularly change learning environments and provide person- or family-centred care to individuals, which can be both physically and mentally challenging. It's important to be able to recognise your own health needs and develop supportive and coping mechanisms. Nurturing your own health and wellbeing will enable you to have the capacity to undertake your academic workload to the best of your ability as well as deliver safe, effective, and high-quality care to individuals when on clinical placement.

TWEET
@PUNC21D

Hello! It's important to me to have a good work/life balance. However it can be hard to achieve it due to study/work constraints and trying to be around for family.

During your time at university, you will be required to manage your own workload and timetable as adult learners. When you begin university, this can be overwhelming and challenging at times; however, implementing coping strategies to manage your time early in your career will enable you to develop and maintain a work/study life balance. This may take a little time to manage at the beginning of your course; however, it's important to seek support early on from your personal tutor/course leader or university support services if you find time management or organisational skills challenging.

What things do you think will help you to maintain a good work/life balance?

_____

_____

_____

_____

_____

_____

_____

At the beginning of your course, you will be given key documents – an academic course calendar and a timetable for your modules. To ensure you are on track and up to date with your studies it's important to plan your time effectively as well as be organised. Utilising these two documents will enable you to plan ahead. For example, recognise when you need to prioritise time to study for an exam and meet with university support networks such as study skills to what time you need to leave to get to class on time.

Your study and personal time will become precious and at times will be varied and hectic; therefore its good practice to use a diary. This can either be a paper or an electronic one. If you are using an electronic version it's helpful to have a paper copy backup – What if you lost your phone or left it at home?

As soon as you have your timetable, ensure to write in your diary your tutorials, classrooms, assignment dates, and shift patterns. You may also wish to consider a wall calendar. This can help you identify important dates for the year/months ahead at a glance such as exams, assignment date, or the start of placement.

Being organised with the course requirement/expectations and a clear overview of your commitments for study/placement will enable you to prioritise and manage your personal life.

When you start your course, you will be given a university email address. Good practice is to check your emails regularly to ensure you keep up to date with any university events or notifications from university staff. See below some helpful tips to email etiquette (Fig 1.3).

Email Etiquette

For students

Writing a professional email may not sound like a big deal, but it's actually a skill in itself

Greet your contact properly
- Include a greeting! It can be as simple as "Dear Dr. Smith," or "Hello, Mrs. Carter," Only use first names IF the person introduced themselves in such a manner. Otherwise use a FORMAL title like Dr., Mrs. or Ms.

Use real words
- Don't use text speak or lots of slang in your message – keep it professional.
- Txt spk mks ur msg hrd 2 read nd on look rly unprofesh!!!

Be polite
- Always remember to say "please" and "thank you" as necessary throughout the email. Instead of demanding be thoughtful and polite. If you are upset about something give yourself some time to calm down and relax so you don't say something you may not actually means to say. *You catch more flies with honey...*

Be brief, positive, and friendly
- Anyone you email may be busy, so make sure you aim for short and sweet. Portray a friendly tone and give options if necessary to show you are willing to work with the other person.

Proofread your email before sending it
- Look over your message for any grammar or spelling mistakes that stand out. Check for tone and make sure your concern is addressed correctly.

Figure 1.3 Email Etiquette.

You may have also joined extracurricular groups or engage with social media. Whilst these digital platforms enhance your student experience and are endorsed, it is important to ensure you maintain boundaries with these platforms to support and maintain your work/study life balance. You may wish to consider engaging with these platforms during certain hours or limit the amount of time you spend on them to enable you to spend time on other wellbeing influences.

As mentioned, the management of modules and placement can be busy, meaning it is important to step away from your course. All aspects of your life can quickly become consumed by nursing; therefore, it is essential to ensure your own identity and passions with your chosen career are met and maintained to reduce the risk of becoming burnout.

Wellbeing and self care

The concept of wellness has been explored and discussed for many decades (Fig 1.4); however, wellbeing can be considered the ability to appropriately respond to expected and unexpected stresses in order to be healthy, happy, and prosperous in work and in life. The Nursing and Midwifery Council – The Code (2018) also recognises the importance of wellbeing and identifies Registered Nurses, Midwives and Nursing Associates should uphold to:

NMC recognise and respect the contribution that people can make to their own health and wellbeing

The NMC code is also very clear that registrants need to ensure that they are healthy enough to practice:

NMC

THE CODE SAYS

20.9 maintain the level of health you need to carry out your professional role

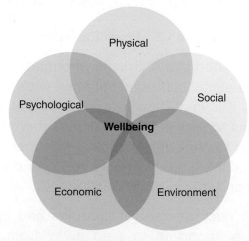

Figure 1.4   Concept of Wellbeing and self care.

Wellbeing can be viewed as a balance between psychological, social, and physical resources versus psychological, social, and physical challenges. Whilst you are studying it can be challenging to maintain a balance of all your wellbeing needs; however, it's important to pause at times to reflect upon your own physical, emotional, and mental wellbeing.

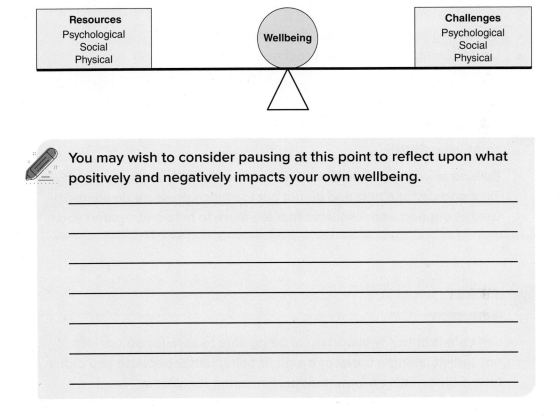

You may wish to consider pausing at this point to reflect upon what positively and negatively impacts your own wellbeing.

_____

_____

_____

_____

_____

_____

How do I maintain my wellbeing?

The World Health Organization's (WHO) guidelines on self-care interventions for health and wellbeing (2022) defines self-care as 'the ability of individuals, families, and communities to promote their own health, prevent disease, maintain health, and to cope with illness and disability with or without the support of a health worker'.

As a nursing student it is important to recognise and manage your own health care needs as well identify support required from others. Below are some suggestions as to how you may enhance your wellbeing during your studies:

- Undertaking physical exercise
- Ensuring healthy eating habits
- Undertaking a hobby's such as crafts, reading, or music
- Exploring the great outdoors
- Having a bath
- Volunteering
- Spending time with friends and family
- Undertaking mindfulness practices

TWEET

@natasha_RMN5

Be kind to yourself and ensure you incorporate self care into your day. Take one day at a time and do not put too much pressure on yourself - use the support and resources that are there to help and support you.

TWEET

@dtbarron

self care is critically important in being able to care for others - it's not selfish taking a break or a sign of being better because you didn't take a break - it's an important part in caring for others.

Within the image below you can see numerous contributing factors on which to improve and maintain self-care. As discussed, at times during your studies it may become busy due to clinical activity, workload, or assignments; however, it's vital to ensure you embed positive self-care needs within your lifestyle to maintain a healthy balance (Fig 1.5).

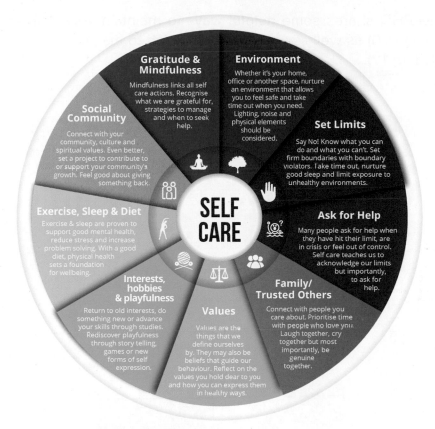

Figure 1.5   **Self Care.** From Betterridge, C. (2018) Self Care Wheel for the Suicide Prevention Workforce. Suicide Risk Assessment Australia, Sydney.

What self-care influences do you wish to embed into your lifestyle and how often?

_____

_____

_____

_____

_____

_____

_____

@BelivePHQ shares some helpful ways to maintain your daily mental health (Fig 1.6) as well as some ways in which to manage stress at university (Fig 1.7).

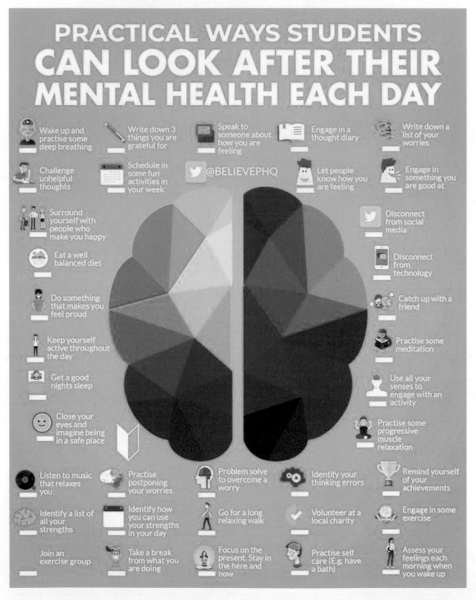

Figure 1.6   **Practical ways students can look after their mental health each day.**

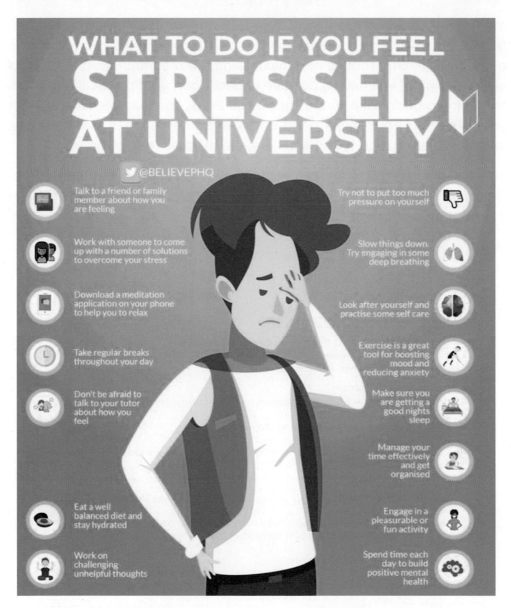

Figure 1.7   What to do if you feel stressed at the university.

As nursing students, you will undertake clinical placements which may include day and night shifts. This may be a routine that is new to you and one which may take a while to get used to. As well as preparing healthy meals for breakfast, lunch, and dinner during your shift, ensuring an effective and meaningful sleep routine is vital for your wellbeing. Adopting a healthy bedtime routine and maximising the recommended 8 hours of sleep per night will have a positive impact upon your physical and mental ability to undertake studies or clinical tasks. You may wish to consider your sleeping environment and consider some changes. For example, invest in blackout curtains/blinds, an eye mask, or ear plugs.

The Royal College of Anaesthetists (2022) have produced some infographics and tips to aid your sleep routine as part of their fight fatigue information pack (Figs 1.8 and 1.9).

 TIP

USEFUL TIPS TO AID SLEEP

In order for sleep to occur, there needs to be deep relaxation. Focus on this first. Deep relaxation is very restorative. Sleep should follow, but if it doesn't, don't worry. Here are some tips that might help improve your sleep.

Unchallenge your brain
- The absence of light stimulates melatonin release; invest in an eye mask and blackout blinds or curtains.
- Avoid using electronic devices for **30–60** min before bed.
- Eliminate unwanted sound with earplugs.
- Consider listening to a podcast or hypnosis audio on a gentle volume to help you fall asleep.

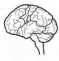

Have a hot bath
- The drop in temperature the body undergoes after a hot bath or shower aids the onset of sleep.
- Bed socks encourage peripheral vasodilation and can help optimise body temperature. Keep your room cool and your bed warm.

Sleep in a way that works for you
Before the existence of artificial light, natural sleep was in two distinct phases, with a break of several hours in-between. Not everyone manages to sleep for a solid **8 hours**; it's what's right for you that matters.

Be prepared
Here are some suggestions to help reduce anxiety and cognitive load, facilitating relaxation.
- Exercise regularly, but not too close to bedtime.
- Download a yoga nidra or meditation audio and use it.
- Write a 'to do' list rather than inevitably thinking of one as you try to sleep.
- Accept help with tasks you can delegate.

Figure 1.8   Useful tips to aid sleep.

TIP

WORKING WELL AT NIGHT

Before nights
- Make sure you usually have a good sleep routine.
- Get extra sleep before your shift. An afternoon nap is ideal as it reduces the length of time you have been continuously awake. A lie-in is an alternative.
- Plan how you will get home. Is there an option other than driving?
- Will you need to rest before driving home?

During nights
- Keep well hydrated and eat healthy snacks. Calories on nights DO count; they contribute to the adverse health effects of night working.
- Maximise exposure to bright lights in non-clinical areas.
- Breaks are essential: Work as a team to cover each other for these.
- A **15–20** min nap can significantly improve alertness.
- Longer naps may result in sleep inertia.
- Be vigilant for the 04:00 dip: Your lowest physiological point.
- Work as a team to check calculations and be aware of the effects of fatigue on decision making.
- If you can, a consistent routine during shifts can help.

Between nights
- If you are too tired to drive, have a short nap before leaving work.
- Have a snack before sleeping so you don't wake up hungry.
- Go to bed as soon as possible to maximise the amount of sleep you will get.
- Do not plan deliveries or daytime activities for the days between night shifts. Warn your housemates that you need to sleep.

Recovery after nights
- Have a short sleep in the morning and then get up.
- Aim to go to bed at your usual time; avoid a long lie in the next day.
- You'll need at least 2 normal nights sleep to reset your sleep routine.

Figure 1.9   Working well at night.

Consider reflecting upon your current sleeping environment. What changes will you make/adapt to ensure you have a healthy sleeping routine?

Everyone at some point experiences challenges with their wellbeing. Therefore, please do not feel you are alone. If you are experiencing challenges in relation to your wellbeing at any point during your studies, please reach out to others who will be able to listen and support. These networks may include:

- Personal tutor
- Course leader

- Practice supervisor
- Practice assessor
- Academic assessor
- University wellbeing support services
- General practitioner

REFLECTIVE PRACTICE

Reflection enables the assessment, evaluation, and learning from a situation which aims to facilitate a deeper understanding of your actions, emotions, and decisions which may inform future practice. The Nursing and Midwifery Council actively supports the engagement in reflective practice, and this is also endorsed by the revalidation process (The Royal College of Nursing, 2022).

NMC The Code is central to the revalidation process as a focus for professional reflection.

The benefits of reflection are:

- Professional development and lifelong learning
- Professional requirement (The Nursing and Midwifery Council)
- Service and quality improvement/public expectation
- Patent safety enhancement
- Linking theory to practice
- Enables practitioners to care for self as well as others' wellbeing
- Supports and enhances resilience
- Facilitates clinical decision-making

The ability to reflect also increases the ability of:

- Self-awareness: knowing one's emotions, strengths, weaknesses, and impact upon others
- Self-reflection: managing one's emotions in different situations
- Increases motivation: facilitates the development of an action plan to improve self/practice
- Encourages empathy: reflecting upon other's thoughts and feelings

- Manage relationships: sharing of reflections can improve multi-disciplinary team working

There are many ways in which you can undertake reflection, some of which are undertaken by yourself or with others such as your personal tutor/practice supervisor or assessor. These can include:

- Written reflections
- Group reflections
- Debriefs
- Clinical supervision
- Reflective journal/blogs
- Schwartz rounds

Undertaking reflection provides you with an opportunity to focus upon self, wellbeing, and emotions. Reflection can be challenging as it requires you to critically evaluate yourself and your performance; however, as it identifies, it can have impactful advantages to self and others. When undertaking reflection it is advised that you use a reflective tool such as Gibbs (1988), Johns (1995), or Driscoll (2007).

YOUR STUDENT VOICE TO INFLUENCE CHANGE WITHIN UNIVERSITY

When you start university, you are entering a community, not a school. In a community, people have a shared attitude and interests in common. You will be working with peers and staff who will all have that common goal of being able to achieve to the best of their abilities. Not only do these opportunities enhance the student environment for everyone, but it also creates opportunities for personal development. Practising your teamwork, communication, and leadership skills can be a valuable experience that will benefit you as a future Registered Nurse.

The university is full of opportunities to work in collaboration with others, whether it would be working groups, research, projects, etc. As an active learner, the only way you can make opportunities happen is to create them. But sometimes, to create the things we want we need guidance and support. This is where university staff can be so useful. Key members of your university journey include:

- Personal tutors/academic assessors – these individuals are the most important to get acquainted with. They are your guides and your personal support aids who can offer you a range of resources to initiate personal and professional development.
- Course leaders – course leaders have an oversight of how the nursing course curriculum is run. They regularly communicate with module teams and students to ensure that the course is running without any issues. Your voice can be powerful if you feel the learning environment can improve.
- Module leaders – you will experience multiple modules throughout your training, each of which will generate different learning outcomes to achieve. Each module is run by lecturers who have developed the module and ensure a module runs smoothly. Module leaders are great individuals to communicate specific module-related concerns, as well as providing feedback on the teaching material.
- Student union representatives – these are a mixture of student and staff representatives who are there for you. They are there to provide support if there are any issues affecting your ability to study.

Please do not view lecturers as a form of hierarchy that wants to control your learning experience. Lecturers are professional peers that can provide much needed guidance on how you want to see yourself within the university environment.

Influencing change through feedback

During your time at university, you may be asked to provide feedback by academic staff, your union, or UK-wide questionnaires as examples. Higher education institutes will actively seek feedback to ensure they listen to students' voices about their university experience which will enable universities to adapt and enhance aspects that impact upon the student's journey. Engaging with staff can be done in a variety of ways, whether it is in person or through feedback processes. All universities pride the voice of students; it is the only way universities know what is going well and what is not going well. Methods include:

- Module evaluations – these are critical to allow modules to address anything that might have impacted the learning environment or highlight things that went well.
- The National Student Survey (NSS) – this national survey opens in your final year of study, and it asks questions in relation to your overall university experience, which includes availability of teaching material, effectiveness of feedback, encouragement of students to succeed, etc.
- Face-to-face meetings – whether on an individual or group basis, your voice is important to drive change. If you do not tell the university about issues or things that have gone well, then the university can never develop.

Contributing to the university

Whilst your voice is important to allow the learning environment to be as engaging as possible for everyone, your active contributions can also bring benefits to the university, as well as yourself. Every university is keen to involve students to not only increase the profile of the university but also encourage opportunities for each student to better themselves. Such opportunities can include:

- Voluntary or charity opportunities – each university often raises money for chosen charities and often puts on fundraising or volunteering opportunities to help a charity. Don't forget, if you have another charity in mind, don't be afraid to do something to help raise money.
- Being a student union representative – this is a great opportunity to work with your peers and to listen to their concerns. By working with the Student Union, you can encourage change that might make a huge difference to all students.
- Getting involved in university projects – universities often have projects that help to enhance the university experience. It is worth keeping an eye out for these opportunities and getting involved.

- Getting involved in research projects – different universities will have different research focuses/themes, so not only will looking for opportunities to contribute to research help the university, but it will also give you valuable insight into research which is vital in nursing.

TWEET
@PUNC20_Michelle

'Im a PALS leader at uni and not only does it improve my own leadership skills and confidence, it allows me to help encourage and mentor out first year.

Think about how you could get involved with things going on in your university

_____

_____

_____

_____

_____

_____

_____

LIVE WELL IN STUDENT ACCOMMODATION

Student accommodation can be a source of stress for many nursing students. Are you planning on going to a university away from home or are you staying close to home? If you are staying close to home, bear in mind that universities will prioritise students from further afield places in student accommodation and therefore you may not get a place in student accommodation.

Think about where you will be living whilst at university and the impact that this may have

_____

_____

_____

_____

_____

_____

_____

TWEET

Keavy Mclean@xkeavy_mcleanx

'I chose to stay at home, I think it's amazing that we have Birmingham Children's Hospital near us! Glad I can have my family support, I wasn't that bothered about moving away'.

"The university I wanted to go to be my local University due to its reputation. I didn't want to spend money on accommodation when I could live at home. I did find that I needed to make more effort to join in social activities to make the friendships I might have if I was staying in accommodation, but I didn't mind. I was quite thankful to return home after a busy day at placement to dinner and knowing I didn't need to worry about washing!"

Universities will have a selection of accommodation halls for you to view and select; the key is to go and look around them. You need to feel comfortable staying there.

- How far is the accommodation from the University campus?
- Are there food shops nearby?
- What are the public transport links?

- What is the security like – consider the flat, building, and surrounding campus?
- What facilities are there on site?
- How long is the contract? Nursing courses are often longer than other student courses and therefore accommodation contracts can finish before terms.
- How much does it cost to live there?
- Who will I be sharing with?
- Are the bathrooms shared or ensuite? Do you have a preference?
- Do you need parking? If so, what are the options?

Please remember to contact your accommodation providers should you have any additional questions.

The legalities of living in accommodation

You will be asked to sign an accommodation contract, so as with any contract take the time to read it. This will contain all the important information around the rights and responsibilities of both yourself and the 'landlord' (it is a two-way relationship) which will be the University or Private company. Hopefully you will not need to refer to it; however, in the circumstance that you do you need to know what you have signed and agreed to.

With many accommodation halls in or nearby city centres holding large numbers of students with arguably predictable movements, it is vital that you get content's insurance. Your accommodation provider may offer this; however, you need to establish this. This will cover several situations such as theft, loss, breakages, floods, and fires.

'Research has found that over a third (36%) of students don't have content's insurance, with many assuming it's too expensive or that they won't need it. But with approximately the same proportion of students falling victim to theft, it's evident that the one-off expense is worth it.' Cheap student contents insurance – save the student (Butler, 2022).

FINANCES

How are you going to afford this? University is expensive but there is help to access. The financial assistance offered by both the UK Government and Universities is ever-changing. You will need to do some research to discover what you are eligible for whilst studying.

Some questions you might need to ask to establish finances to support your university accommodation include:

- What are the eligibility criteria? Everyone has a different set of circumstances and these influence what we are entitled to
- When do you need to pay for accommodation and when is the bursary, grant, or loan paid – is it at the end of a term ready for the next or is it at the beginning of the term? This will help you plan your finances
- Establish whether the financial support is a bursary, grant, or maintenance loan. Ensure you read the terms and conditions carefully
- Is the amount you are entitled to means tested?
- How much are you eligible for – this is key to helping you identify if this helps cover the accommodation
- How do you apply – universities and the government will have timeframes to receive your financial applications? Ensure you check the deadline dates, and be prepared and organised on this; you don't want to miss the opportunity

ACCESSING SUPPORT

Attending university is tough but equally can be life changing. There will be times you need additional support, and it is important that you do to ensure you continue with your studies. Nursing courses are notoriously known to be challenging as you are juggling academic work with clinical placement and outside life.

TWEET
@KatSuffolk

'Students think support is not for them or is hard to do'

TWEET:
@LauzPUNC2019

'See if your University has a writing café/maths group to help improve your writing and try and go to the writing café a couple of times before the deadline'

TWEET
@emilyoc_

'If you don't get through to the person you were trying to contact, keep trying other people until you get the support you need'

The support universities have is for every student to access at any time. Please reach out if you need help; there are many people and support systems that can help you. You are not alone.

The NMC set out expectations that universities have such support in place.

NMC

THE CODE SAYS

3.13 are provided with information and support which encourages them to take responsibility for their own mental and physical health and wellbeing

3.14 are provided with the learning and pastoral support necessary to empower them to prepare for independent, reflective professional practice

The university you attend will have support systems that you can access.

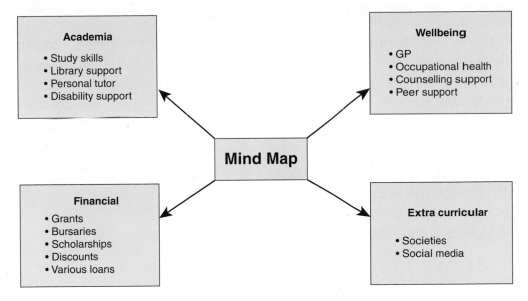

Do not underestimate your student union! You will probably become acquainted with where the Student Union Bar is on campus; however, there is so much more to the support system offered. They can signpost you to lots of different support inside and outside of the universities, support you with writing statements.

Think outside the box – social media is a great and powerful way to access support from nursing students and Registered Nurses who are or have experienced situations you too will be. Many students find this online platform particularly useful because they feel reassured they aren't alone and support problem solving. When you are out on placement you will have additional support to draw upon such as your practice supervisor, assessor, placement area, and education team. They all have experience in supporting students and have a wealth of knowledge.

UNLOCKING POTENTIAL – EMOTIONAL AWARENESS

Our brains go through a process when learning new skills and knowledge, combining two different functions of the brain: the unconscious part and the conscious part. Sigmund Freud, a famed psychoanalyst, coined the phrase 'unconscious mind', the part of our mind that houses aspects and factors that are not in our control.

The goal we strive for is to be at least consciously competent, having awareness and confidence to recite what we have learned. This allows us to be more confident in critically thinking about topics or solving problems. Ideally, we want to be unconsciously competent in which we do skills without even thinking (Fig 1.10). How we learn is highlighted below (Burch, 1970):

1. Unconscious incompetence
2. Conscious incompetence
3. Conscious competence
4. Unconscious competence

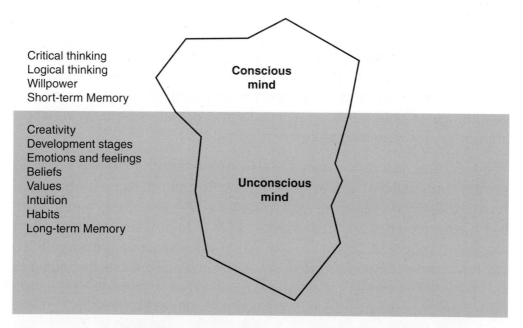

Figure 1.10   **The differences between the two types of minds are often illustrated as an iceberg. (Freud, 1915).**

If you have ever learned to drive a car, you will remember that at the very start you were very aware that you did not know how to change gear. Now, you probably don't give any thought when changing gear – this is unconscious competence.

This conscious awareness of our abilities is influenced by unconscious factors developed from our life exposure. For example, some people will be consciously aware that they are not competent in physiology knowledge. Unconscious factors are built into our mindsets by how we were raised, how we were educated, experiences with life events, etc.

Part of the unconscious mindset are emotions, triggered by neural or hormonal physiological mechanisms in response to events. Emotions are different to feelings; emotions are energy flowing through our body. How we feel is our conscious mental interpretation of the emotion, and it might differ from person to person. How we interpret an emotion influences our way of thinking towards a task, which can impact performance on a task. This is shown in a model presented by Dr Alan Watkins (2012) (Fig 1.11).

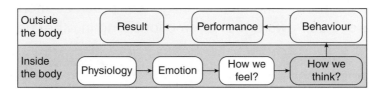

Figure 1.11   Interpret an emotional influences.

How our brains are wired to deal with the physiological mechanisms will differ from person to person. Some people might be more sensitive to mechanisms like the fight or flight response due to life exposure, something we can't control. This can reflect on how we interpret emotions such as fear.

It is ok to feel anxious, frustrated, or sad when facing difficult tasks. But the reality is that the way we interpret emotions will change the way we behave. If someone is feeling anxious, for example, and they interpret anxiety in a negative way, they will likely have low morale which will affect their performance. But we can tap into the physiological mechanisms and take back some, if not complete, control.

There are always two choices to deal with different interpretations of emotions, whether positive or negative. Acting on it is ideal as we will learn, but sometimes we are not ready, so walking away and reflecting on the situation is ok too. Both are active strategies that promote healthier association with your emotions.

For example, during exams you might feel nervous or anxious, which increases your heart rate. This increase in your heart rate overwhelms and switches off your frontal lobe of the brain (where your logical ability is), making your brain more 'foggy'. Mindful breathing lowers your heart rate, which will improve your brain's performance.

Feeling uncomfortable about certain situations is a way of life; we cannot avoid this. Only by pushing outside our comfort zones can we learn how to deal with situations and increase our personal toolkit that helps our wellbeing. It doesn't matter whether you have an introverted or extroverted personality; if you increase your emotional awareness and understand how they change your attitude and behaviour to situations, you will improve your performance, unlocking your potential.

The four domains of emotional intelligence, provides more ideas on how to improve self-awareness of emotions, and in other people:

Self-awareness	Self-management
• Do not view emotions as good or bad. • Don't be afraid to branch out your comfort zones. • Learn and reflect on your values in life. • Notice the impacts your emotions have. • Use books, films, or music to help recognise emotional responses. • Ask for feedback. • Learn how you respond to stress. • Keep a daily journal. • Recognise when emotions affect you physically.	• Take time to breath. • Share your goals and aspirations. • Ensure you have a good sleep pattern. • Stop focusing on your limitations. • Identify someone who helps as a self-manager. • Schedule time for things you enjoy. • Smile when you can. • Learn to identify emotion from reason. • Accept that there are situations you cannot control. • Learn something new from everyone you meet.
Social awareness	Relationship management
• Identify and learn particular body language. • Live in the present moment. • Greet people by their name. • Look at the whole picture (think of the iceberg). • Read the room and understand the mood. • There is nothing wrong with just listening. • Clear away any clutter. • Don't take notes when you know information will be provided at the end of a session. • Imagine yourself in the other person's shoes.	• Remember small things make the big things happen. • Feedback should be specific, direct and constructive. • Don't be afraid to show how much you care. • Create space for people to talk to you. • Respond positively to feedback. • Work to build trust. • Be open and curious. • Enhance anger into something positive. • Don't meander around difficult situations. • Avoid quick fix answers that do not benefit others.

The advice provided is only effective when you must deal with situations outside your comfort zones. If the way you feel is affecting your day-to-day life, then please speak to your GP or your personal tutor. Mental health disorders can have a devastating impact on your wellbeing and may require interventions such as counselling or medication.

UNLOCKING POTENTIAL – CHANGING YOUR MINDSET

How we view failing or not passing tasks can link to what has been discussed when looking at optimising personal performance. Often, many people have a negative association with failing, implying it is a direct reflection of their abilities.

Some of you may fail an assessment during your nursing journey, but it does not mean you are not good enough. Failure is learning: do you really think NASA worked out how to go to the moon straight away? It took a lot of mistakes and failures to get NASA to where they are now.

Things like academic writing is a skill that many will be good at right from the start, and for some it will take time to improve, and that's ok. You are all going to take different journeys to achieve what you want, so some might need additional support to achieve a goal, and this is also ok.

We need to embrace our individuality and not feel threatened by those who may seem to have a better grasp of a challenge; their circumstances might be different to yours. So, how we view failure will be different because of our experience with failure in our pasts. This builds an established set of attitudes which drive how we think and act on failure, a mindset.

Dweck (2016) introduced two different mindsets: a growth mindset and a fixed mindset. A fixed mindset is a set of attitudes that accepts ability is fixed, whilst a growth mindset is a set of attitudes that embraces growth and challenges (Fig 1.12).

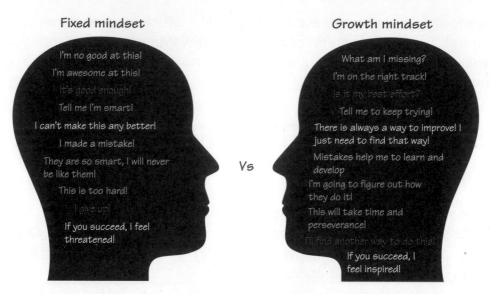

Figure 1.12   Picture shows key differences between a fixed and a grow mindset. (Dweck, 2006).

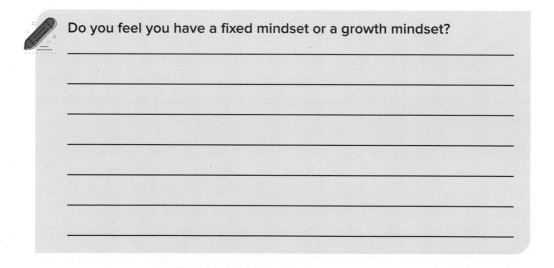

Do you feel you have a fixed mindset or a growth mindset?

_____

_____

_____

_____

_____

_____

Life is full of challenges, and it can be scary. But whilst most of the time challenges can be difficult to overcome, they are opportunities for personal development. You might overcome a challenge the first time, or you might need to reattempt until you achieve what you want.

These steps can allow you to change your mindset based on the principle of growth mindset (Dweck 2006).

- Accept you are unique: accept that you might take things at a different pace to others. Your focus is on your development, not how others want you to be.
- Let go of a desire for things to be perfect: whilst it might seem that pursuing perfection is proactive, for someone with a fixed mindset it can act as a shield, acting as a barrier to growth.
- Embrace lifelong learning: appreciate that there are opportunities everywhere to learn more; our minds are curious and want to learn all the time.
- Let go of the need for approval: don't focus on needing approval or appreciation for what you have done; focus on self-development.
- Rethink how you feel about failure: mistakes are necessary for us to see what we need to develop; otherwise, we will never improve ourselves.
- Just add 'yet!': if you ever think, 'I can't do this!' Or 'I don't know this!' Just add the word 'yet'. It's amazing how something that small can make such a big difference.
- Don't be afraid to come out of your comfort zone: just think what's the worst that could happen if you try something different.
- Face challenges in the present moment: don't view challenges based on what has happened or what might happen. Take every challenge in the present moment, and deal with the outcomes as they come.

How to seek advice and support to help personal/professional development?

Feedback from assessments is designed to help you improve your academic skills, not highlight that you are not good enough. So, it's always good to seek support on how to improve your academic ability:

- Reflect on the feedback. Analyse the feedback and write down the areas that have been highlighted.
- Be aware of your emotional responses. Remember, previous experiences can dictate how you respond to feedback. Recognise these and look at things from a bigger picture.

- Seek support from your marker. Come up with at least three questions or ideas on how to improve your assessment. This will make a tutorial more proactive.
- Seek support from your academic assessor/personal tutor at university. They will be aware of services that might benefit you.
- Access peer support groups to help you see different perspectives.

CONCLUSION

This chapter aimed to explore how to make the most of your time at university. It's an exciting time to start university and your nursing career and we hope you enjoy your journey. Starting and adapting to University and nursing can be challenging at times; however, through this chapter we have explored ways you can look after yourself as well as signpost you to support networks. We wish you all the best for your journey ahead.

Now you have finished this chapter. Please make notes on what you have learned.

_____

_____

_____

_____

_____

_____

_____

_____

_____

_____

_____

_____

_____

_____

_____

_____

_____

_____

_____

_____

REFERENCES

Butler, J. (2022). *Student Contents Insurance 2022*. Save the Student. Student contents insurance 2022 - Save the Student https://www.savethestudent.org/accommodation/student-contents-insurance.html.

Dweck, C. S. (2006). *Mindset: The new psychology of success*. New York. Random House.

Goleman, D. (1995). *Emotional intelligence*. New York. Bantam Books, Inc.

Holt, J. (1984). *Growing without Schooling*. Volume 40. Boston. Holt Associates.

Donna (2021) https://twitter.com/Punc21D/status/1448726941671043090?s=20&t=cRym0K3Pvf9zNhUd4QMDDw.

Natasha. (2022). https://twitter.com/natasha_RMN5/status/1526645037131497477?s=20&t=cRym0K3Pvf9zNhUd4QMDDw.

Nursing and Midwifery Council. (2018). *The Code: Professional standards of practice and behaviour for nurses, midwives and nursing associates*. https://www.nmc.org.uk/standards/code/. [Accessed 23 September 2022].

Royal College of Anaesthetists. (2022). *Fight fatigue resources*. Online. https://anaesthetists.org/Home/Wellbeing-support/Fatigue/-Fight-Fatigue-download-our-information-packs. [Accessed 23 September 2022].

Royal College of Nurses. (2022). *Revalidation requirements: Reflection and reflective discussion*. Online. https://www.rcn.org.uk/Professional-Development/Revalidation/Reflection-and-reflective-discussion. [Accessed 23 September 2022].

Ted Talks. (2012). *TEDxPortsmouth – Dr Alan Watkins – Being brilliant every single day* [Part 1]. https://www.youtube.com/watch?v=q06YIWCR2Js. [Accessed 21 September 2022].

DRISCOLL, J., 2007. Practising clinical supervision: A reflective approach for healthcare professionals. 2nd ed. Edinburgh: Elsevier.

GIBBS, G., 1988. Learning by Doing, A Guide to Teaching and Learning Methods. London: Further Education Unit.

JOHNS, C. (1995), The value of reflective practice for nursing. Journal of Clinical Nursing, 4: 23-30. https://doi.org/10.1111/j.1365-2702.1995.tb00006.x

Freud, S. (1915). The Unconscious (Standard Edition, vol. 14, pp. 159-190). London: Hogarth.

The Obama White House. (2009). *President Obama's message for America's schools.* https://www.youtube.com/watch?v=8ZZ6GrzWkw0&t. [Accessed 12 September 2022].

World Health Organization (WHO). (2022). *WHO guideline on self-care interventions for health and wellbeing, 2022 revision.* Online. https://www.who.int/publications/i/item/9789240052192. [Accessed 23 September 2022].

TWITTER REFERENCES

Barron. (2022). https://twitter.com/dtbarron/status/1192538178235904002?s=20&t=cRym0K3Pvf9zNhUd4QMDDw.

BelievePHQ (2022) https://twitter.com/BelievePHQ/status/1525055775005106176?s=20

Cotter, M. (2022). https://twitter.com/PUNC20_Michelle/status/1570779461481824259?s=20&t=n7YuRDzPBs-f2E5Sm3jnaA.

Lames, H. (2018). *There is a huge value on having your practice watched and receiving feedback for improvement in patient safety and experience as well as your own professional development.* https://twitter.com/hannahlames1/status/954089676314431488?s=20&t=cRym0K3Pvf9zNhUd4QMDDw. [Accessed 21 September 2022].

Laura. (2022). https://twitter.com/LauzPUNC2019/status/1562452885895401473.

Mclean. K (2022) https://twitter.com/xkeavy_mcleanx/status/1570768919497179136 accessed September 2022.

O'Caroll, E. (2022).https://twitter.com/emilyoc_/status/1562476888966443008.

Suffolk, K. (2022). https://twitter.com/KatSuffolkSTN/status/1562405229785751552.

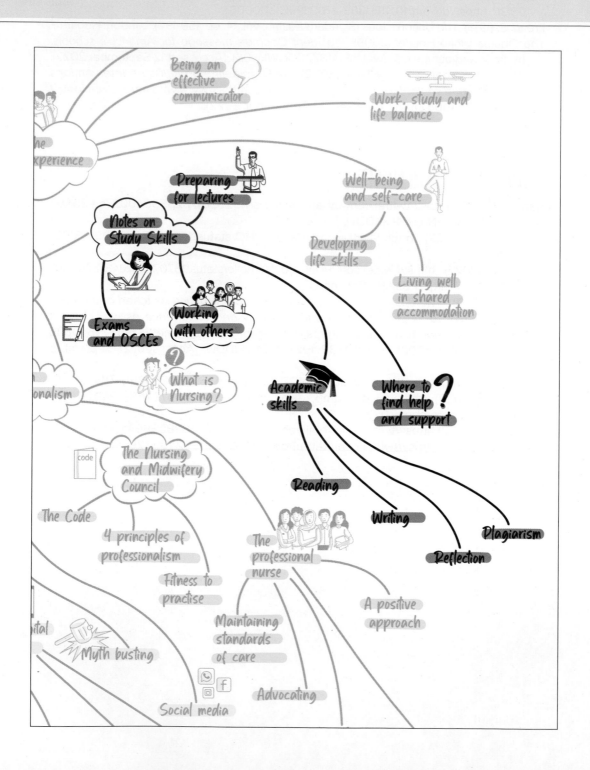

NOTES ON STUDY SKILLS

Christie Roberts (She/Her)

INTRODUCTION

Some of you may have come to university straight from school, or some of you may have taken a break from study and are now returning. Whatever your circumstances are, it's important to remember that this is your journey – so you can take charge and make it your own!

As part of your nursing course, the NMC expects you to undertake 2,300 hours of theoretical study to complement the clinical learning that takes place. Therefore, it is important to start off on the right foot. University learning is likely to be different from any other learning that you may have done before, as the responsibility lies with you to make it successful. It can be daunting entering the university environment for this reason; however, you will develop skills, knowledge, and personal attributes that will serve you well in life – such as the ability to prioritise your workload, control over your own learning, and critical thinking, to name a few, which are also important nursing skills! But to be successful, you need to be able to use your time effectively and find ways to keep motivated when times are challenging.

Self-efficacy, or being able to manage yourself, can make a significant difference to your time as a student and even into your nursing career. It is one of the most important attributes to develop during your studies; therefore, it's worth spending some time thinking about this and developing your self-management abilities. The more you engage with your course and actively seek out ways to enjoy learning, the higher the likelihood that you will not only survive the experience but thrive. This chapter aims to help you to understand the university environment, the expectations for academic work, and aspects of skills required for academic work and to help you explore yourself as a student.

What are your immediate concerns about the academic environment?

_____

_____

_____

_____

_____

_____

_____

UNIVERSITY LIFE

What can you expect a typical week at university to look like? Well, it is likely to be the equivalent of a full-time job (for full-time courses), around 35–40 hours. However, not all this time will be spent in a classroom; it will be a mixture of lectures, tutorials, independent study at home or in the library, and on placement.

- Lectures: these vary greatly but usually involve listening in large groups. Some expect participation or flipped learning and there might be recorded sessions. Flipped learning means that you attend prepared, having covered some of the material before you start. This allows for more effective listening as you already have some knowledge about the topic before you attend your lecture.
- Tutorials: these are used to give feedback on your work and to guide and discuss your progress. It's important to arrive prepared and create an agenda or list of questions about what you want to ask during your attendance. If you are hoping for feedback on your work, be prepared to discuss what you think it means and why you received it.

- Seminars and workshops: involve group discussions, can include student presentations, set reading, guest speakers, or lecturers.
- Independent study will likely consume most of your week. It requires good time management and strong motivation.
- Group work or collaborative learning could involve discussions, projects that form part of your final grade, or peer support.

Preparing for lectures

Whether they're happening online or face-to-face, some preparation during your theory blocks in university is needed to stand a chance of following along and to help you get the most from the learning. Given that approximately 50% of the course is spent doing theory, through larger group lectures and smaller, more interactive seminars, it's important that you know how you can best get yourself ready through independent study. Your theoretical knowledge is essential for building proficiency in nursing, alongside your clinical experiences.

> 'Theory offers what can be made explicit and formalised, but clinical practice is always more complex... Theory, however, guides clinicians and enables them to ask the right questions'.

> *– Patricia Benner*

Many universities will upload learning materials that will be used onto your online learning platform ahead of time. Looking at these prior to lectures to familiarise yourself with the content can help you to keep up with whoever is delivering your session and allow for more effective listening. This can be particularly useful for people who do not speak English as their first language, and people who have dyslexia or other accessibility needs. Your university will also upload or send you any additional reading or pre-session activities that you'll be expected to complete, so it's essential to give yourself time to go through this. It can be tempting to skip some of the independent learning, as there is no one telling you that you need to do it, but on nursing courses you get out what you put in and you'll get a lot more from the teaching if you've taken the time to prepare beforehand.

Set aside enough time before a lecture to go over any relevant resources. This may include skim-reading articles, watching videos, reading book chapters, or taking quizzes to assess what you already know.

You may realise that you are already familiar with some of the content and may find areas that are new which require further research. It's also a good opportunity to think about any questions that you may want to ask during your lecture or seminar.

You may feel more comfortable working from paper than a screen, so consider printing any resources out and having them available to annotate during teaching sessions. The same applies to note taking before or during lectures – notes can be typed or handwritten depending on what you find easiest and quickest, and this will vary for every individual. According to the poll below, people tend to prefer handwritten notes, but there are also many people who find electronic versions more convenient. Make the most of highlighters or different colour fonts to identify the key information, and consider including visuals like pictures, diagrams, or mind maps to boost your understanding of a topic.

TWEET
@christienursing

Student nurses of Twitter! What's your preference when it comes to writing notes for lectures, seminars, pre reading etc? Any top tips you'd like to share about note taking? What works for you, what doesn't? @StNurseProject @RCNStudents @WeStudentNurse #SuccessfulStN

Hand written	66%
Typed/electronic	34%

TWEET
@B_Swiff_

'I downloaded the PowerPoints prior and [there] is an option to leave notes at the bottom [of] each slide. Very effective. Generally just use Word- saves doing the same thing twice. I find IT much better than paper!'

TWEET

@LouHyettC

'I print the lecture slides and then make notes directly on them during the lecture. Then afterwards, simplify/bullet point my notes into mind maps and write my own MCQs for revision'

Many courses use a 'spiral curriculum' across the years of teaching – (Fig 2.1) this means you'll be revisiting and revising similar topics and theories each year but going into more detail each time to reinforce and expand on learning. This can also incorporate Benner's seminal 1982 'novice to expert' model. This means having notes that make sense to you, and that you can easily refer back to, can be a huge advantage when building on existing knowledge.

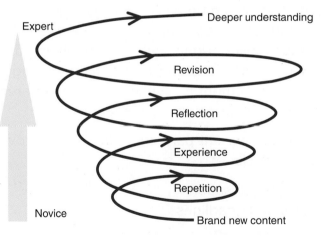

Figure 2.1 Spiral curriculum.

After each lecture or seminar, it's worth taking the time to go over your notes again to ensure you've understood everything that's been taught. Take this opportunity to look up any new terms or unfamiliar concepts, do some further reading around a topic, and research anything that you found interesting or surprising. This may generate further questions that you can ask your peers or tutors and help with the absorption of new information.

TIP

Creating multiple choice questions (MCQs) to quiz yourself and/or your peers can improve retention of new information and boost active recall.

If you do have questions, don't be afraid to ask them – you're probably not the only one thinking about it. Soon after the lecture is a good time to ask them, as the topic is fresh in your mind and your lecturer's mind.

Organisation and time management

During theory blocks, it can be easier to organise your time as there is more structure and routine compared to living around placement shifts. Aspects like childcare and regular activities that help you maintain your work-life balance, such as exercise and socialising, might be easier to schedule. Time management is a vital skill for Registered Nurses, and this can be developed during your time at university.

There are lots of component parts that contribute to overcoming procrastination. These include:

- Planning and organisation
- Setting goals and deadlines
- Prioritising tasks
- Eliminating distractions
- Rewarding yourself
- Taking adequate breaks

There are various organisational tools that can be utilised for general time management. These include wall planners, diaries, online calendars, and scheduling apps. They allow you to visualise important dates and deadlines in the context of any other responsibilities. For example, it can be particularly difficult to keep track if you have academic deadlines that fall during a placement block, so having these highlighted can help you maintain your awareness of upcoming due dates and keep on top of allocated shifts.

Lots of students find that time blocking helps them to maintain concentration on tasks without getting distracted or starting to procrastinate.

'I like to set aside an hour to work on my essay. When that hour is done, I move onto something else, like research for placement or watching something on TV. Means I don't end up wasting time because I'm trying to force myself to work for a longer time when I've lost focus. I usually do that a few times throughout the day so I might end up only working on my essay for like 3 hours, but they're productive hours because I don't feel burnt out'.

– Thea Gibbons, nursing student

The Pomodoro method can also be used to manage time – dividing your available time into 25-minute blocks with a 5-minute break in between. This can help to boost productivity, reduce procrastination, and avoid multi-tasking by promoting focus on the task at hand for shorter periods of time. Alternatively, you might want to commit to a 'power hour' to work intensely for a longer period. Some people may find that once they start working and get into a rhythm, they just want to keep going until they run out of steam. Take some time to establish what works most effectively for you.

You can maximise the time available by taking quiet opportunities to do any reading or independent study – for example, if you commute to university or placement on public transport, you may want to use this time. However, you should also remember to take enough breaks away from studying or researching and allow yourself enough time to step back from learning, take a break, rest your eyes, and give your brain and body a chance to relax and think about something other than nursing.

'In my first year as a nursing student, I was all over the place. Didn't know how to study properly, didn't know how to take a break. I'd done a previous degree but the difference in workload in nursing, and mixing it with placement and practical sessions, really threw me. I would spend hours copying out notes but nothing would actually go in so it felt like a huge waste of time because I'd have to go over the same notes so many times. I kept on doing that for basically all my first year and honestly really burnt myself out for the start of 2nd year. It got so bad I considered taking some time out of uni but decided to carry on and just really prioritise figuring myself out, like how, where and when I work best, and working on self care so I could go into final year and feel like I was doing my best before I qualified'.

– Ash Khair, Registered Nurse

If you're really struggling to get going and find you're just staring at a book or a screen for hours on end without taking anything in or making any progress, take some time out. It might be that the format of the information isn't the best format for you, or that it's not the best time of day for you to engage with academic work in a constructive way. It may be that you're not in the right headspace at that time – maybe you're hungry, or tired, or overwhelmed? A change of environment can be beneficial in shifting brain-blocks, so a 10-minute walk and some fresh air might be all you need to get going again. Regardless, you don't need to beat yourself up and try to force it if you find that productive study isn't happening naturally.

Creating a focused to-do list at the start of the day can be beneficial in goal setting and prioritisation of tasks. The psychological evidence for making lists includes improved concentration and reduced anxiety through structure and control of your goals (Masicampo and Baumeister, 2011; Maio, Haddock and Verplanken, 2019). Importantly, your to-do list should be realistic for what you can achieve in the time available. You probably won't be able to write your assignment from start to finish in a day, but if you divide it up and allocate time for other essential or pleasurable activities, you can get a much clearer picture of what is attainable.

To Do List

Thursday 01 September

- ☐ Write essay introduction
- ☐ Write essay 1st paragraph
- ☐ Call the dentist
- ☐ See Sarah for coffee- 2pm
- ☐ Webinar- 7pm
- ☐
- ☐
- ☐
- ☐
- ☐

If you find that you're getting distracted by your phone, there are lots of apps and tools available that can block social media sites or stop you from using your phone at all:

- Forest plants a tree that grows over the length of a timer you've set – using your phone during that time will kill your tree.
- Freedom blocks social media and other internet pages so that you're unable to access them whilst you're trying to focus.
- The Do Not Disturb function on your phone can stop distracting notifications from popping up.

If you get distracted being in your own house, either by other people or by the environment, try somewhere else. The library is good for people who might get side-tracked by conversations but might not be ideal if you don't work well in a quiet environment. Group study spaces within your university or cafes could be better if you want to work collaboratively and have conversations whilst working.

Self-management

Self-management is about knowing what works best for you – and this might take a little while to figure out as it is different for everybody.

Take some time to consider what you already know about your best ways of working and note these down below. Consider things such as:

- The time of day – Are you a night owl or a morning lark? Can you pull all-nighters? When are you least likely to be busy with other tasks?
- The study environment – Do you get distracted being at home? Does the library or a coffee shop work better? Is it helpful to have other people around?
- Motivators – Would you rather start and finish early, or is the upcoming deadline a motivator for you? Do you have something nice planned for afterwards that can keep you going?
- Music choices – Classical music works for some, pop music works for others. Do you prefer to work in silence?
- Individual learning styles – Does watching a video or listening to a podcast work better than reading an article? Can you remember information better if you're reading it aloud to yourself or to other people? There's more information about learning styles below if you're not sure what works best for you.

If you're not sure about your preferred learning style, the VARK model can help to give you an idea. VARK stands for **V**isual, **A**uditory, **R**eading/Writing, and **K**inesthetic (Fleming and Mills, 1992) and knowing how you work best can help you shape your self-directed learning so that it's more efficient and effective. You can fill out a quick questionnaire on **vark-learn.com** that can help you think about your learning style and what methods work best for you. It's worth trying out a variety of methods until you know what feels best for you. Some suggestions are listed below:

Visual-	Auditory-
• Charts, diagrams, graphics • Images with or without labels • Visually appealing/ colourful resources	• Videos • Podcasts • Collaborative work • Talking things through out loud • Repeat to a friend • Verbal instructions
Read/write-	**Kinesthetic-**
• Books and articles • Written instructions • Write and re-write • Printed handouts and PowerPoints • Note taking	• Simulation and role play • Hands-on activities • Tactile • Live training sessions • Presentations

'I realised during first year that I'm most productive at night and would often only start working at 11pm. During theory blocks this was fine but wasn't feasible whilst I had placement shifts starting at 7am, so I had to change my timings and make the most of days off to catch up on academic work'.

– Christie Roberts, nurse

Work-life balance

All work and no play can rapidly lead to burnout. This is true for nursing students and is true for Registered Nurses, so it's a skill that's worth developing now. Maintaining a work-life balance can require conscious effort for nursing students, particularly when you're on placement full time, juggling academic work, and are somehow expected to also see your friends, look after your family, or take part in clubs and societies. It is hard, but not impossible, and definitely important.

> *'Plan fun things to look forward to for any down time (straight after exams/placements)'.*
>
> **– Kerri Smith, nursing student**

Having something to look forward to can act as a motivator if you find you're struggling to keep the end in sight. Having weekly scheduled activities like an exercise class or socialising can also provide you with a regular, designated time when you don't have to think about uni.

Some students may also be working part time alongside studying – this can make it more difficult to establish a work-life balance but may be necessary for your personal finances. If this applies to you, it is important to make sure that you've still got enough time to rest and to allow as much time as you'd like for university commitments, as ultimately, this should be the priority. It will be worth having a conversation with your manager about your hours to reach a consensus about what is feasible to work in the context of your other responsibilities and deadlines. Consider if you can self-roster your shifts/hours or look at jobs with a casual/0-hours contract which will allow you to pick your own hours without a minimum monthly requirement.

It's important to remember that your schedule might look vastly different to someone else's schedule. No two students are the same, and you can't expect that anyone will manage their time or manage themselves in the same way as you – you can be totally unique in your approach to academics at university! People may have different commitments and responsibilities outside of the course, so it's important to stick with what works for you and your personal situation and preferred ways of working.

ACADEMIC SKILLS

Reading and note taking

Reading and taking notes form the foundation of academic success at university. To gain confidence, it is important to know what to do and how to do it. Which of these beliefs do you think is true?

- You need to read everything on your reading list
- All books should be believed

- All journal articles must be read from beginning to end
- Good notes should look good

Well, the answer is none of these are true. Let's explore further:

You need to read everything on your reading list: One of the main differences between reading at university and reading at school is at university you have autonomy over what you choose to read, which means it is likely you will be reading different texts from your peers, even if it's all for the same assignment.

When it comes to reading to inform your academic work, quality is often more important than quantity. A few high-quality sources that inform a balanced argument will often serve you better than reading every available book and article, which may just leave you feeling overwhelmed and no more informed.

All books should be believed: Another difference is that you are expected to read beyond the words on the page, think critically, and determine for yourself if the text is important, why it's important, and how it relates to other text and ideas.

At university, you are expected to adopt an active approach to your studies. This means that instead of passively reading and noting things down, you need to engage your brain and think about the information before, during, and after reading and making notes. This means you will be able to develop your own informed views rather than memorizing what the text says.

All journal articles must be read from beginning to end: How much you need to read from an article will depend on why you are reading it – you don't have to read an article in full if you're just trying to get a feel for key themes in a subject area and can skim-read several articles or read the abstracts more quickly to gain an overview. If you are trying to find specific information and details, then more focused reading may be necessary.

By reading every article cover to cover, you're likely to be taking in a lot of extra information that you won't actually find helpful in your studies. You'll need to use your judgement when deciding which sections of a resource you'll need to read. For example, just reading the results section won't give you any insight into why the research was carried out, or if the research is high quality.

TIP

Never judge a journal only on its title. Read the abstract of the journal article to gain a better idea of what the paper is about. You should be able to tell fairly quickly if this will answer your assignment question. You could also read the recommendations and conclusions too. At the very early stages of the course, you need to have some knowledge of methodologies but don't allow this to weigh you down.

Good notes should look good: What constitutes good notes will be entirely individual for each student. Good notes don't need to be aesthetically pleasing, just clear enough that you can read, understand, and absorb the content. Your individual learning style will influence the notes that you write – for example, visual learners may include more images and diagrams in their notes compared to auditory learners, who may prefer notecards that can be more easily read aloud.

The 'spiral curriculum' was mentioned earlier, and your notes will be a vital resource when it comes to revising and reviewing past information to build on existing knowledge.

Writing

In your first year, academic work will be graded at Level 4 (A-Levels, BTECs and Access courses are equivalent to Level 3). This will increase up to Level 6 by your final year, so you can expect to see progression in the expectations of your academic work, reflected in marking criteria or grading rubrics – this may seem daunting, but you'll simultaneously experience progression in your personal academic skills as you move through the course which will allow you to keep up with the development.

Academic writing at a university level may feel very different from academic writing that you've undertaken previously, but it builds on existing skills such as structuring your writing, using appropriate grammar, and constructing clear and concise sentences. Academic writing uses the third-person voice. Instead of saying 'I' or 'we', you would use an impersonal style – for example, saying 'this essay explores...' rather than 'in this essay, I will explore...' or 'research has demonstrated...' instead of 'I have found that...'. The exception to this rule is in reflective pieces of work, where you may be writing in first person language. Sentences should not be so long that the reader gets lost or loses focus midway through. Generally, one sentence will cover one point – but relevant additions could be joined by separating the sentence with a dash or semicolon.

> *'Do not write so that you can be understood, write so that you cannot be misunderstood'.*
>
> *– William Howard Taft*

Most pieces of writing will follow the same structure:

 TIP

Introduction

Do what it says on the tin – you're going to be introducing the essay. This is a place to outline any aims and objectives for your work and provide background or context as to why you're including certain aspects. It should be concise and signpost the reader to the layout of the essay and it generally won't be greater than 10% of the total word count. It might seem counterintuitive, but it can be easier to write the introduction at the end once you know what shape the assignment has taken.

REMEMBER: Aims are broad statements outlining what you want to have achieved by the end of your assignment. Objectives are more specific statements outlining the steps that need to be taken to get to a measurable outcome, or how you're going to achieve your aims.

Body of text

This is the bulk of your work and should take up most of your time and word count. Each paragraph will usually be covering a separate point and should be supported by fully referenced evidence. The 'PEEL' acronym can be used to help with paragraph structure – first you make your **P**oint, then introduce your **E**vidence, provide an **E**xplanation, and **L**ink it to the next paragraph. Paragraphs should flow logically from one point to the next and you might find that reading your work out loud can help you decide if any reordering is needed.

Continued

TIP—cont'd

Finally, there shouldn't be too much variation in the sizes of your points in the main body of text; if one point only takes a few sentences and another takes up half a page, review whether you can split the bigger point into more focused sections that may be easier to read, and consider finding additional information or resources for the smaller point (if there's nothing else you can think to say about it, maybe it doesn't even need to be included?). Reading your paragraphs aloud is a good way of assessing how well they flow and connect.

Conclusion

Your final paragraph should not be introducing any new information and should not contain any references, as you are simply summarising what has already been said. Alongside providing a brief overview of your key points, you should be considering whether you have answered the assignment question or fully addressed the essay title throughout your work. Like the introduction, this ideally will consist of 10% of the total word count.

REMEMBER: In-text references will count towards your total word count, but your final reference list and any appendices will not.

Academic writing should be backed up by the body of evidence available, and a key theme in writing at a university level is demonstrating that you've moved past the face-value meanings of research, evidence, and concepts and are not just describing these but that you have begun to think critically (more about that later) and have considered why these things are, what the implications are, or why it's important.

One way of achieving this is by avoiding direct quotations – repeating the information verbatim doesn't demonstrate that you've understood the information or data beyond the words on the page or have assimilated the deeper meaning into your writing to develop your argument. Where possible, aim to paraphrase any sources you use and combine information with other sources that contribute to the point you're making (this might also include introducing sources that disagree with your point, if there is conflicting evidence).

TIP

If used, direct quotations should have the page number included as part of the in-text citation, if available.

In some assignments, you may be given more flexibility in regard to the focus of your essay — for example, choosing a specific condition to focus on, or exploring a particular aspect of nursing practice. Although this can feel daunting as there's a wider scope of things you can choose from, it does give you greater creative licence when it comes to writing your essay. It can be useful to make a list or mind map of any direction that appeals to you and make brief notes about what you could include. You could consider things that you've covered in university, resources that you're aware of, experiences from clinical placements, and any other personal knowledge. You will find it easier and less laborious to research and write about if you can pick an area that you actually find interesting and engaging.

'When you can, choose topics that genuinely interest you so it makes writing about it easier'.

– Kerri Smith, nursing student

You may be given an opportunity to submit a formative assignment before your final, summative work is due. The style of formative opportunities can vary — for example, submitting a plan of your essay, a first draft, or the initial few hundred words. It's recommended to take the opportunity for formative submissions where possible as it can give you a rough idea of what whoever is marking your essay is looking for or can guide the focus of your work (ideally before you go 2,000 words in the wrong direction!).

Once you've finished writing, it can be tempting to submit your work and get it 'out of sight, out of mind'. However, taking a moment to proofread and edit can help pick up minor errors, including spelling, grammar, and references, which can impact the overall quality of your work and gain you a few vital, extra marks. It's recommended to take some time away from your work before you proofread so you can come back to it with fresh eyes. Although spellcheck will pick up on most queries, it shouldn't be trusted 100% of the time – for example, it may not pick up on issues like using the wrong version of 'their', 'there', and 'they're', as they are all technically correct. Reading your assignment backwards can work as an alternative to focus on the technical aspects of your writing without getting distracted by the content. Alternatively, you could ask someone who doesn't know as much about the subject area to read it and provide comments on details like conciseness and paragraph/sentence structure.

Each university will have different requirements for formatting and submitting academic work, so make sure you are familiar with any specific requirements and clarify any expectations. These may include:

- Anonymous submission using a student number rather than your name.
- Attachment of a departmental coversheet or any other relevant documentation.
- Double line spacing.
- Specific fonts/font sizes.
- Allowances for word counts – some institutions may allow you to be to 10% above or below the specified limit.

For further information, enquire if your university has any resources on academic writing, or reach out to your subject librarians for assistance.

Evidence-based practice – appraisal and critique

The NMC requires that Registered Nurses 'always practice in line with the best available evidence' (NMC, 2018, p. 10)

NMC

THE CODE SAYS

6 Always practise in line with the best available evidence
To achieve this, you must:
6.1 make sure that any information or advice given is evidence-based, including information relating to using any health and care products or services

But how do you know what the best available evidence is? As mentioned, not everything that is written in books, journals, or any other source of evidence should be believed, and not everything is a high-quality source of information – therefore, it shouldn't be taken at face value without further consideration of its strengths and weaknesses.

The process of appraising the quality of evidence will involve thinking critically about what you've read and questioning the research. Things to consider when critically appraising research and evidence:

- What type of evidence is it? Where does it fall in the hierarchy of evidence?
- Where has it been published? What is the impact factor of the journal?
- Has the article been peer reviewed? This is where professionals in the same field will evaluate the article prior to publication and make suggestions for improvements or changes – this process improves the quality and validity of the work.
- Are the authors credible and qualified in their field? Have they previously produced work related to the topic?
- Is the information still relevant? Could it be out of date? Have there been any significant developments in the field since it was published? Is it a seminal or highly influential piece of work?
- What is the aim of the evidence? Who is it aimed at – Patients? Professionals? The public? Why is it being discussed or researched?
- What are the strengths and limitations of their research methods? How is the research being conducted and is it the most appropriate technique? Consider sample size, sampling method, data collection, and data analysis.

- Are there any ethical issues, biases, or conflicts of interest? These should be declared at the beginning of the article.
- Do other sources confirm or deny the findings presented? What are the key themes in the wider body of evidence? This will introduce wider reading around the subject area. Consider using the reference list of the article as a starting point to identify additional relevant research.

TIP

The International Academy of Nursing Editors has produced a directory of credible journals, which is available on their webpage.

It can be overwhelming to try and think about so many aspects of critical thinking, but there are various frameworks for appraisal that you'll learn more about during your course. If you are new to critical analysis, the 'Six Questions for Critical Thinking' tool (Aveyard, Sharp and Woolliams, 2015) is often recommended as it provides a simple structure for those just beginning to think about thinking critically. Having a clear list of criteria that you use to consider evidence means that you can approach it more systematically and are less likely to miss any steps out.

Phrases that relate to critical analysis of evidence include:

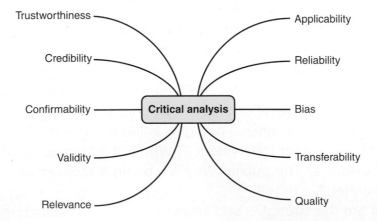

Failing to think critically about published evidence can have real-world implications.

CASE STUDY

In 1998, Dr Andrew Wakefield had a paper published in *The Lancet* describing a link between children receiving the MMR vaccine and the onset of autism. Due to *The Lancet* being seen as a highly credible journal, these findings were widely shared with little consideration of the study itself – vaccine scepticism and subsequent measles outbreaks were noted. Following the investigation and presentation of multiple studies demonstrating no credible link between vaccination and autism, the paper was retracted in 2010 and Wakefield was found to have acted unethically, with misrepresentation of data and deliberate fraud when conducting the study and publishing his results. For example, lying about recruitment methods, falsifying or omitting data when it did not fit predicted findings, and failing to disclose financial conflicts of interest in the study (Rao and Andrade, 2011).

Some students find that the evolution and development of critical appraisal can be one of the biggest expectations whilst moving through your nursing course, so it's worth taking the time during first year to start building your confidence and begin integrating it into your academic work. There are lots of books available which outline critical thinking skills and tools that can structure your analysis of evidence.

TWEET

@karolinaviolet:

'Moving your brain on from overly descriptive language to critical analysis! That was a tough one and I love the theory side of the course. Personally, number one tip: make sure you have access to plenty of nursing research/critical thinking/evidence appraisal books'

High-quality evidence forms only one part of evidence-based practice, alongside professional judgement and patient preference or values (Aveyard and Sharp, 2017) but it is essential to ensure that you are providing safe, effective, and informed care to patients in clinical practice.

Social media

Social media can provide an excellent platform for learning. Twitter, as an example, hosts lots of 'tweetorials' and educational threads that can provide knowledge from experts in their fields. Similarly, you can find lots of quizzes, blog posts, and account takeovers on Instagram on a variety of nursing and healthcare topics.

Remain aware that there are no checks for credibility and validity on social media. Be cautious of the accounts you're following and the information you're receiving – apply your critical thinking skills!

Referencing

'When a thing has been said and said well, have no scruple. Take it and copy it'.

– Anatole France
(As long as you fully cite your source...)

Referencing is the process of acknowledging any sources you use – everything from articles, books, videos, webpages, interviews, and more. Referencing is necessary as it allows statements, facts, and claims made in your writing to be substantiated and demonstrates that you have recognised the words and ideas of others within your work and are not claiming them as your own original thoughts. There's no fixed rule for how many references should be included in a piece of academic writing, but you want to make sure your entire assignment isn't just a patchwork of other people's words without any of your own synthesis or analysis. As a guide, 1 reference per 100 words is generally acceptable (so for a 2,000-word essay, you'd be considering 20 references as a benchmark). There may be key sources that are introduced during your lectures or that are featured on your module reading list that can act as a good starting place for information and that you may be expected to reference within your work.

Each university will have a specific referencing system that they would like you to use (if you're not sure what you should be using, ask!) and may provide a guide with information and examples, but every system has an in-text reference, usually in the author-date style, accompanied by a full citation in the reference list at the end of your work. The information required for each entry in your reference list will depend on the type of source, so make sure to check your referencing guidance to make sure you've included everything – and pay attention to punctuation and italics. Reference lists should be listed alphabetically (Microsoft Word has a function that will sort this for you, rather than organising your list by hand).

TIP

'et al.' translates to 'and others' and is used when there are multiple authors. You may need to reference each author initially but usually can then switch to *et al.*

Completing your reference list as you write, rather than leaving it until near the end, is recommended as it means you can quickly and easily identify any sources you've already used and reduces the fear of your internet browser suddenly shutting down and losing any sources that you've been using which you hadn't cited yet.

'During an assignment where I didn't update my reference list for days and just wrote the in-text citations, my computer shut down and I lost every webpage that I had open. It took hours to try and re-find all the sources that I had used, and after that I made sure to complete my full reference as soon as I included the source'.

– Christie Roberts, nurse

It's up to you whether you cite your sources manually or using referencing software. To name a few, websites such as 'Cite This For Me' and 'Refworks' can generate references electronically dependent on the information you input and will keep a list of references for you in a bibliography. Google Scholar also provides references in a range of different styles – look for the 'cite' button underneath the article on the search page. Please remember that they may not provide the reference

100% accurately and it is worthwhile double-checking before you submit your essay. If you're really stuck on a particular citation, it's worth asking a librarian, as they may be able to help you pick out and format any specific information.

Plagiarism

Failure to reference your sources appropriately can be considered plagiarism, whether it was intentional or not. Software used by many universities for submission of assignments, such as TurnItln, can generate a numerical value of comparability, referred to as a similarity or originality score, and will highlight in your submission where these comparisons have been made. The system produces this by comparing your work to thousands of sources including webpages, articles, and work submitted to the same system by other students. There is no universally agreed value for an acceptable similarity score, but there is some leeway to account for things such as the essay title or any essay cover sheets that will match work submitted by other students at your university. Direct quotations, even if fully referenced, will also increase the score – but this wouldn't count as plagiarism as long as the source is properly credited, and the words are presented in quotation marks. Whoever is marking your essay should take these things into account, particularly if your similarity score comes back on the higher side.

 TIP

Put your pen or keyboard out of reach. Read the article you are using and then cover it up. Write, or type, the key concepts of the passage in your own words.

It is possible to plagiarise yourself if you use parts of your own previously submitted assignments. To avoid this, make sure you are not lifting sentences or paragraphs from older essays, and fully reference any sources that are used. If you are working on assignments collaboratively with peers, it's also important to make sure you're not accidentally plagiarising each other or producing work that is too similar. It can be useful to discuss academic concepts or sources with others, but you should not be working together whilst actually writing or preparing for final submissions due to the risk of plagiarism.

In a worst-case scenario, plagiarism amounts to academic misconduct and can have huge impacts on your progression through the course – but it's easily avoided by making sure you're not directly copying others' work and are including accurate citations to indicate that you have used someone else's ideas, words, or research to inform your own work.

EXAMS, OSCES, AND PRESENTATIONS

Many students will cite these aspects as the most nerve-wracking during their university course – but this doesn't need to be the case! Your preparation for these assessments will be a key determinant of your performance and can help to reduce the anxiety associated.

Exams

The key to preparing for exams is fundamentally having the information in your head, ready to be used when needed. This doesn't mean the information should just be memorised. Memorisation of information means you're likely to be able to recognise the information required but potentially not be able to actually *remember* it and be able to use it effectively – not helpful for exams, or for your longer-term development. Instead, you should focus on a technique called 'active recall' – a technique that focuses on retrieving information from your brain instead of passively putting information into your brain.

Tools that can be used to help with active recall include creating mnemonics (for example, OLDCART for pain assessments), using flashcards with definitions to be matched to terms, and developing your own multiple choice questions (MCQs) that you can use to test yourself or others. Testing yourself will also highlight any gaps in your knowledge that require further revision.

TIP

1. Work on your exam mindset. Being aware of negative thought patterns and feelings will make a huge difference in exam preparation. Try replacing negative thoughts with ones more constructive.
2. Revise with others: form a study group with some of your peers. This is a good opportunity to ask each other questions and test and quiz each other, and of course, it provides a bit of encouragement and motivation!
3. Create a realistic revision timetable that you will stick to.
4. Don't wait until the exam period to start your revision – create them as you go through your modules.

OSCEs

OSCE stands for 'Objective Structured Clinical Examination'. Fundamentally, it's a practical exam that could test clinical skills such as communication, medication administration, A to E assessments, and more.

Given that it's a role-play-based exam, role play will probably be the most effective way to prepare. Try creating groups of three to act out practice scenarios – one as the Registered Nurse, one as the patient, and one as an observer to make notes and check against the marking criteria. Recording yourself practising can also allow you to critique your own performance and pick up on areas for further practice. There may be videos available that outline the skills that you're being assessed on, so watching these might give you a starting point for what your examiners are looking for. When asked what markers are looking for, here is what they replied:

TWEET

@Laura_Jane278:

'I am just looking at how you behave in practice. I'm not just looking at the clinical skill, but your whole interaction and your professionalism. Ultimately, if I was that manikin, how would I feel on the receiving end of that care contact?'

TWEET

@CYP_UoB_Kelvin:

'Clear and obvious proof you have performed the required task. Clear communications- speak clear and confidently. Be professional- adhere to uniform requirements and be professional. Ensure you perform the fundamental tasks- it could make or break your OSCE'

During the exam you might feel nervous or uncomfortable – so fake it till you make it! You might not feel confident, but nobody else except you will know that. Things like open body language and loud and clear speech will help you relax into the scenario and give you an air of confidence.

TWEET

@nursingnoodle:

'Talking as someone who failed & had to repeat the module over one year, it is absolutely not something you can do without practice, in fact, more than you think is necessary even if you're sure you know it! It's SO daunting but I actually found it great for my learning. Find someone to practice with- whether it's someone on your course, a friend, or partner. Repetition helps. I used dry wipe pens on laminated copies that would be used in the OSCE'

TWEET

@sam_thomas02:

'If you don't already, learn to talk to yourself! I found speaking through exactly what I was doing and why I was doing it really helped me to prepare! Also agree re find a study buddy and do a "mock" OSCE beforehand'

Presentations

Similar to OSCEs, the best way to prepare a presentation is by practicing in conditions mirroring real life — saying it out loud, to an audience, in a defined time frame, and with any slides or presentation aids that you intend to use. It can help to ask your audience for feedback on aspects like the speed of speech or clarity of your voice.

If presenting as part of a group project, make sure you've practised it as a group at least once before the real thing. Make sure you're all aware of who is covering which sections and the order that you're speaking in. You'll also want to make sure that you can get through the presentation in the allocated time, considering that people may speak faster or slower than usual when nerves kick in.

When it comes to the topic of your presentation, it's preferable to have a narrower but deeper area of focus compared to a wider topic. This will help you to have a more manageable amount of content to cover within your time limit. If you're using a PowerPoint presentation alongside, aim to have minimal writing on your slides; this means people will be able to focus more on what you're saying rather than spend the time reading lengthy slides. Finally, it's okay to have prompts on notecards, but try to minimise how much you're relying on these whilst you're speaking. The delivery of your presentation will seem more self-assured and fluent if you're able to look out at the audience rather than down at your notes.

Again, you might feel nervous presenting to a crowd but try to remember that your peers in the audience or anyone else presenting in your group will probably feel the same. If all else fails, try to picture the audience in their underwear!

REFLECTION

Reflective assignments provide the perfect place for you to critically examine your experiences and to consider what went well and what you would change next time. Generally, these pieces of writing will be less objective, and evidence driven and will be more descriptive and emotive. As you are writing more personally, reflective essays will usually be written in first-person language and may not include as many references as a standard assignment – although they will contain some, as it is still an analytical piece of writing. Including relevant evidence can also help to link theory and practice.

'I think initially I didn't understand the importance of reflection in nursing as it wasn't explained to us very well in first year, however now as I'm at the end of third year, reflection has been really useful, it's helped me to breakdown complex situations that I was unsure about and how different actions could have changed the situation'.

– Becky Lowe, nursing student

Using a framework will provide guidance for what to include in your reflection and help you to structure your work. The model that you choose to use may depend on the type of reflection – for example, if you're completing a reflective assignment versus a brief reflection after a good shift or a challenging situation. You'll need to use your own judgement to decide which structure is most appropriate and will help you to reflect most effectively for each individual situation.

Some of the models that you might come across include:

Gibbs' reflective cycle

The Gibbs' model is cyclical and consists of six steps-

1. Description – an outline of the experience, with context for the situation.
2. Feelings – both during and after the event.
3. Evaluation – consider how yourself and others reacted, and how the situation was handled. Was it a positive or negative experience?
4. Analysis – what were the key aspects of the event? Are there any key theories or guidelines that influenced actions?
5. Conclusion – was there a positive or negative outcome? Were there any alternative actions that could've been taken – what would the outcome have been in that case?

6. Action plan – identify any learning points and consider how you will achieve these. How would you respond in a similar situation in the future?

Driscoll's 'what' model

Three quick and simple questions to ask yourself to reflect on a situation:

1. What? Describe the situation, consider what actually happened and how you felt about it.
2. So what? What is the significance of the experience? As a result of the circumstances, what was learnt?
3. Now what? What changes or learning can be implemented? How will this be achieved?

ERA cycle

Another simple, cyclical model with three steps:

1. Experience – either positive or negative. It could be a brand-new experience, or something you have experienced previously.
2. Reflection – how did it go; how did you react, and how did it make you feel? What could be improved upon?
3. Action – how will learning inform future practice? What tools or resources might you need? Your actions will lead to new experiences, and the cycle continues for ongoing learning.

When thinking about what your experience taught you, you may consider incorporating learning objectives or goals from your clinical practice competencies and could also make links to other competencies and the NMC Code – this demonstrates that you have moved past being purely descriptive and into a more critical and analytical viewpoint.

'Writing down brief reflections about both positive and negative experiences allowed me to consider my practice and in particular see how I had developed from my first year to my final year-particularly in more "abstract" ways like my confidence and curiosity, which aren't measurable with competencies'.

– Christie Roberts, nurse

Reflection is a useful skill for becoming more aware of your practice, is essential for lifelong learning, and is also one of the component parts of appraisals and of the revalidation process once you've entered the register (which you definitely don't need to worry about for now – but the NMC website has more information on this and the other requirements). The ability to reflect on situations can help you move past things that were challenging and appreciate things that went well.

GROUP WORK

As a student, you may be asked to work in groups. This can provide some challenges, but it is also an opportunity to develop key skills. As Registered Nurses, working as part of a team will be a daily occurrence, so participating in group work at university will allow you to practise.

How do we make group work work? Most of us will have work as part of a team before we attended university, so it would be useful to think of a previous situation where you work in a group that worked well and ask yourself:

- What made the group successful?
- What skills do you need to develop to work effectively with others?
- What skills do you have that bring value to the group?

When your group is formed, there are some things you can do to make sure it's a success from the very start.

- Get to know each other: it might sound simple, but it will really bring the group together, allowing everyone to understand each other better. It is also worth considering creating ground rules.

_____

_____

_____

_____

_____

_____

_____

- Allocate roles: some roles that could be formed would be a note-taker which will ensure that everyone knows what was discussed if anyone is unable to attend the meeting or forgot what was said. A group chair is also a useful role as they can lead the discussion and ensure that everyone has a chance to speak with no one person monopolising the conversation. If you have a group presentation to produce, there may be someone who is confident with public speaking who could be allocated this role. When allocating roles and tasks, it is a good idea to delegate based on everyone's strengths. There is no point in having someone who is a strong leader be the note-taker. However, group work is also the opportunity to learn and develop skills. For example, if you are shy and hate public speaking, you may see this as an opportunity to practise this skill. Remember: not every task needs to be delegated. There are some situations where working as one team would be more beneficial – such as brainstorming ideas.
- Be organised: decide how you are going to work together as a team. Are you going to meet in person? Are you going to video call? Group chats? Will you be using a shared folder? It sounds obvious, but it will really save any miscommunication.

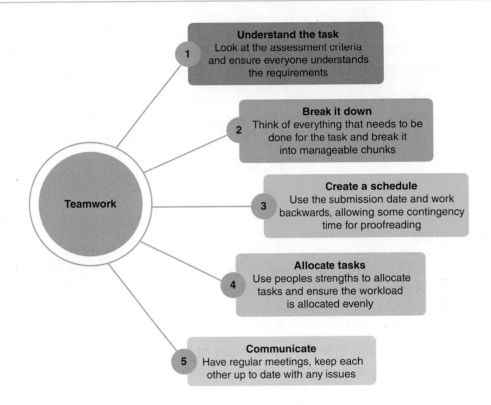

Teamwork

1 **Understand the task**
Look at the assessment criteria and ensure everyone understands the requirements

2 **Break it down**
Think of everything that needs to be done for the task and break it into manageable chunks

3 **Create a schedule**
Use the submission date and work backwards, allowing some contingency time for proofreading

4 **Allocate tasks**
Use peoples strengths to allocate tasks and ensure the workload is allocated evenly

5 **Communicate**
Have regular meetings, keep each other up to date with any issues

'Towards the end of my first year, I created a study group that encouraged me to study in a different way using the Feynman study technique. This involved me choosing a topic I would teach to the group'.

– Aghogho Wanogho, nursing student

TROUBLE SHOOTING

Accessing support

One of the most important things to remember during your university career is that help is always available, as long as you know where to look and when to ask for it, from speaking to your lecturers about course content to accessing student support services for more pastoral issues, to engaging with disability support services for support plans and learning difficulty advice.

Librarians specific to your nursing faculty are also excellent resources, and it's recommended that you identify who from library services is responsible for nursing early on, and don't be afraid to go and say hello!

Peer support can also be vital — it's helpful having people in the same boat. Everyone will have different backgrounds and experiences, and this can make for some insightful, mutually beneficial conversations. Supporting each other often contributes to a more inclusive learning environment where students feel comfortable sharing experiences and asking questions.

Managing expectations

In your first year, there's no expectation that you'll be able to do everything perfectly on the first try. The expectation is that you will try your best, put in the work to prepare for learning, and ask for help when you feel out of your depth. By doing these things, you'll be able to learn and develop your knowledge and confidence. Your expectations for yourself should match these — you won't know everything and sometimes things won't go as well as you hope or expect. All you can keep doing is trying and take note of the moments when you feel proud of yourself and realise how far you've come.

Disappointing grades

At some point during your time as a student, you may receive a grade for an assignment that you're unhappy or disappointed with. The most important thing to remember is that this will probably happen to everyone, and that it's not the end of the world. Try to avoid comparing your results to others — and remember that your educational background, commitments and responsibilities, and personal circumstances will all contribute to your grades.

Almost everyone will tell you that a disappointing result should be seen as a learning opportunity. Your marker should have provided some feedback to give context to your grade, but if you feel that you would like more clarification then reach out to your faculty to gather more feedback and consider areas for improvement more closely.

Remember that feedback is not intended to make you feel bad about your work but instead should be seen as a foundation to improve on – some people may refer to feedback as 'feed forward', as the intention is to help you with your future submissions.

TWEET
@Iona_bluesky:

'Also find out if student services have support. At my university you can have up to six sessions per year to go over work and structure etc. Talk to your lecturer about the work, and other students about their perceptions of the assignment'

Once you've identified the specific areas that you can improve on, start thinking about how to make that happen (spoiler: it probably won't happen overnight!). There are people within your university who can help you with aspects of your academic work, including student support, subject librarians, and disability services. Academia takes an army, and there's no shame in asking for help from those who can provide it. Equally, your course mates can be a valuable resource – maybe there are a few of you that are struggling with a particular aspect, and you could reach out for assistance together or ask your tutors to set up a feedback workshop or tutorial.

TWEET
@PhilBallRN:

'Give yourself some time to look at other things in life. Then seek feedback on the area that led to the disappointment. Find a trusted colleague to help focus the revision or rewrite requires, and be confident of your strengths of which there will be many'

TWEET
@stn_jemma:

'Speak to the module team or marker about what you need to do to improve it, see if there's someone who can read it for you, and don't be too hard on yourself'

TWEET

@Bex_Runs:

'[I've] had to resubmit a LOT. My best advice is, don't let is beat you. You're not a bad person or a failure because you didn't pass first time. Find out where you didn't get marks, then make your work better. It's only in academia where not passing first time is considered failure'

As you can see from these tweets from both nursing students and Registered Nurses, a disappointing grade shouldn't be seen as a personal failure. However, that doesn't negate the fact that it can really hurt to not perform as well as you hoped or expected, or to have not passed an assignment or exam and be faced with a resubmission or resit. Take some time to be disappointed before you start thinking about next steps – often talking it through with someone you trust can help to express your feelings.

If you are required to resubmit an assignment or resit an exam, your grade will likely be capped (this is usually at 40%). You might feel disappointed, frustrated, or upset and this is completely natural – it's not a reflection on your journey through nursing, and remind yourself that you're still learning. You don't need to rush into re-writing (within the confines of the deadline), so take enough time to think through areas for improvement and to consider any feedback before you start and utilise your university team – they are there to help!

CONCLUSION

The academic side of your course is just as important as the clinical practice side, so hopefully this chapter has provided some useful hints and tips to help you put your best foot forward when preparing for teaching, attending lectures and seminars, and working on your assignments both individually and as part of a group. There are many aspects of academia and the university environment which can feel initially overwhelming but try to remember that you won't be the only one feeling this way, and that there is plenty of support available should you need it. Some study skills may be brand new to you, so reflecting on your university experiences can be a gratifying way to see your confidence and skills grow throughout your time as a student.

Now that you have read through this chapter, spend some time thinking about how you plan to develop your self-management ability, including establishing your individual learning style and your time management strategies. Also think about what activities you can incorporate into your week to maintain a healthy work-life balance and consider any resources you may need to keep on top of deadlines and commitments. Remember: this is your journey, so stick with what works for you.

Now you have finished this chapter, please take time to refelct on your learning.

_____

_____

_____

_____

_____

_____

_____

_____

_____

_____

_____

_____

REFERENCES

Aveyard, H., Sharp, P. (2017) A beginners guide to evidence-based practice in health and social care. 3rd edn. London: Open University Press.

Aveyard, H., Sharp, P., Woolliams, M. (2015) A beginner's guide to critical thinking and writing in health and social care. 2nd edn. London: Open University Press.

Benner, P. (1982) 'From novice to expert'. American Journal of Nursing, 82(3), pp. 402–407.

Driscoll, J. (2007) Practising clinical supervision: a reflective approach for healthcare professionals. 2nd edn. Edinburgh: Bailliere Tindall Elsevier.

Fleming, N., Mills, C. (1992) 'Not another inventory, rather a catalyst for reflection'. To Improve the Academy, 11(1), pp. 137–155.

Gibbs G (1988). Learning by Doing: A guide to teaching and learning methods. Further Education Unit. Oxford Polytechnic: Oxford.

Jasper, M. (2013). Beginning Reflective Practice. Andover: Cengage Learning.

Maio, G., Haddock, G., Verplanken, B. (2019) The psychology of attitudes and attitude change. 3rd edn. London: Sage.

Masicampo, E., Baumeister, R. (2011) 'Consider it done! Plan making can eliminate the cognitive effects of unfulfilled goals'. Journal of Personality and Social Psychology, 101(4), pp. 667–683.

Nursing and Midwifery Council (2018) *The Code: Professional standards of practice and behaviour for nurses and midwives.* https://www.nmc.org.uk/globalassets/sitedocuments/nmc-publications/nmc-code.pdf (Accessed 13 August 2022).

Rao, T., Andrade, C. (2011) 'The MMR vaccine and autism: Sensation, refutation, retraction and fraud'. Indian Journal of Psychiatry, 53(2), pp. 95–96.

TWITTER REFERENCE

https://twitter.com/christienursing/status/1564300332582244352?s=20&t=3ntaQldk Nz8XmGJdxutjaw (Accessed 01 September 2022).

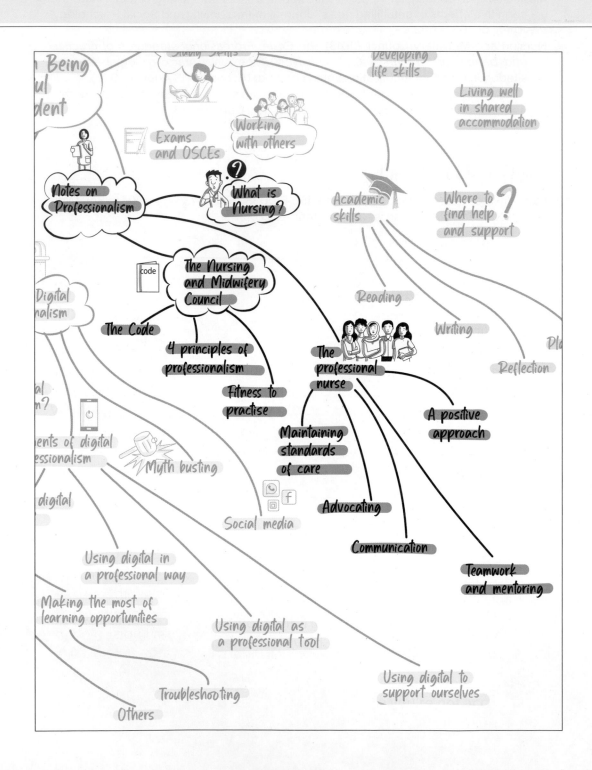

NOTES ON PROFESSIONALISM IN NURSING

Calvin Moorley (He/Him) ■ Joshua Sharman (He/Him)

INTRODUCTION

On enabling students to develop into a professional Registered Nurse. It will cover areas on the Nursing and Midwifery Council (NMC) Code which sets the standards for being professional. In this chapter we explain how regulatory bodies work and their importance in nursing. As well, we explain professionalism and how understanding other cultures and groups contributes to being a professional Registered Nurse and a member of a professional group.

WHAT IS NURSING?

Traditionally nursing has been viewed as a vocation and this concept is rooted in the history of nursing, where religion played an important part in caring for the sick and destitute and nuns often tended to the sick or those requiring care in the community (Capparelli 2005). You may also be more familiar with the history of Florence Nightingale who served in the Crimean war in the 1850s. She attended and cared for soldiers whilst recording the disastrous conditions in which care was being delivered. Nightingale urged the British government to increase resources and was pivotal in improving the standard of care and professionalism in nursing.

Another historical nursing figure who is often overlooked is Mary Seacole. Mary Seacole was a Jamaican-born nurse, who also contributed to the care of soldiers during the Crimean war. Prior to the war Mary Seacole had experience in treating patients with cholera and later yellow fever. She was turned away by the British War Office to help in the Crimean war and funded herself to get there to help care for those wounded in battle.

A key thought is that nursing is to do with caring and looking after people. However, nursing entails much more and has developed from a vocation to a profession; it has a professional regulatory body called the Nursing and Midwifery Council (discussed later in this chapter) and Registered Nurses can gain academic qualifications from BSc to PhD.

WHAT IS PROFESSIONALISM?

Professionalism is the skills, knowledge, and understanding of a job; it is where the individual adheres to a code, standard, and or set of principles (Moorley and Puthernpurakal 2019 in Moorley 2019). These are usually reflected in a set of qualities that reflects the profession the individual belongs to. Professionalism is demonstrated in the way you behave, your attitude, and the ways in which you communicate with others. From the description of professionalism, you can see that in nursing it is more than wearing a uniform, being polite, and looking neat and tidy; however, these aspects should not be dismissed as they contribute to being a professional Registered Nurse. Professionalism in nursing is about possessing and demonstrating a set of values that are critical to patient care and at the same time these values improve the methods, standards, and policies that drive nursing practice.

'To me professionalism in nursing is about my behaviour in person and online, it is about following the NMC Code and demonstrating the values of nursing through caring for patients and their families as well as working with my colleagues in a harmonious way that improves nursing'.

– Sanchia, nursing student

CASE STUDY

Kobi is originally from Ghana and has been living in London for the past 10 years. He has been attending a further education college doing a health and social care studies foundation course. He met a Registered Nurse on one of the college's career days and attended a talk about nursing as a profession and career. He had never thought of nursing as a career, and after doing some research and speaking to his tutors he applied to undertake his pre-registration nursing education. He is now preparing for his interview and has started thinking about what it means to be a Registered Nurse.

In Kobi's interview he was asked what the indicators of a professional Registered Nurse are.

Can you think of an answer that he can construct?

_____

_____

_____

_____

_____

_____

PROFESSIONAL REGISTERED NURSE

When Registered Nurses act professionally, they improve the communication between the team and individual colleagues, patients, and their relatives (Moorley and Puthernpurakal 2019 in Moorley 2019). This leads to increased accountability for practice and a better clinical environment, all resulting in a better care experience for the patient. These are linked to standard 7 (Communicate clearly) and standard 8 (Work co-operatively) of the NMC's Code.

NMC

THE CODE SAYS

7 Communicate clearly

To achieve this, you must:

7.1 use terms that people in your care, colleagues and the public can understand

7.2 take reasonable steps to meet people's language and communication needs, providing, wherever possible, assistance to those who need help to communicate their own or other people's needs

7.3 use a range of verbal and non-verbal communication methods, and consider cultural sensitivities, to better understand and respond to people's personal and health needs

7.4 check people's understanding from time to time to keep misunderstanding or mistakes to a minimum

7.5 be able to communicate clearly and effectively in English

8 Work co-operatively

To achieve this, you must:

8.1 respect the skills, expertise and contributions of your colleagues, referring matters to them when appropriate

8.2 maintain effective communication with colleagues

8.3 keep colleagues informed when you are sharing the care of individuals with other health and care professionals and staff

8.4 work with colleagues to evaluate the quality of your work and that of the team

8.5 work with colleagues to preserve the safety of those receiving care

8.6 share information to identify and reduce risk

> **8.7** be supportive of colleagues who are encountering health or performance problems. However, this support must never compromise or be at the expense of patient or public safety

There are different ways as a nursing student you can demonstrate professionalism which can be built into your practice as you graduate to a Registered Nurse.

Advocating for patients

To advocate for a patient means that you can speak up for that patient's wishes and how they feel. It can happen during a team meeting; when agreeing care plans and care packages; and when liaising with other agencies or healthcare professionals concerning the patient's care. As part of advocacy, you would learn to uphold the patient's rights and act in their best interest, which is also part of the NMC Code standard 4: Act in the best interests of people at all times.

NMC

THE CODE SAYS

4 Act in the best interests of people at all times

To achieve this, you must:

4.1 balance the need to act in the best interests of people at all times with the requirement to respect a person's right to accept or refuse treatment

4.2 make sure that you get properly informed consent and document it before carrying out any action

4.3 keep to all relevant laws about mental capacity that apply in the country in which you are practising, and make sure that the rights and best interests of those who lack capacity are still at the centre of the decision-making process

4.4 tell colleagues, your manager and the person receiving care if you have a conscientious objection to a particular procedure and arrange for a suitably qualified colleague to take over responsibility for that person's care (see the note below)

While doing this you must always remember to act with kindness, show respect, and maintain dignity.

> *'For me, advocacy means speaking up for the patient in my care. I should be able to make known or convey their wishes to the entire team by acting on their behalf. I should be doing this despite the patient's background. To be an advocate sometimes takes courage'.*
>
> **– Eucharia, nursing student**

When advocating for any patient, it is important to take into consideration their background and characteristics such as age, gender, religion, sexual orientation, disability, race and ethnicity, and culture.

These are areas that require particular attention; you may have a patient from a particular religion that prefers to be in a female-only part or bay of the ward. You may find that you have to advocate for a patient with an intellectual disability and may need to take time to ensure you are representing the patient in an authentic way. Sometimes what a patient wishes or wants may be different from their families' wishes, and for them, you may have to advocate for a patient against their families' wishes, and you will need to develop a professional stance with the families when advocating.

In essence, good professional behaviour in advocacy is putting the patient first. Once you begin to advocate for the patient you will realise that this calls for effective communication, verbally and non-verbally.

Communication

It is essential to communicate in any episode of care; this can take the form of both verbal and non-verbal means. Verbal communication involves speaking or using speech to communicate with another individual or group to share information. Non-verbal communication is any form of communication that does not involve speaking. All nursing staff (Registered Nurses or nursing students) should always communicate in a clear and effective manner. An important aspect of professional Registered Nurse communication is that when you are speaking to any patient and their family you speak in a way that they can understand you (e.g. use words that they can understand) and try not to use medical jargon that may lead to confusion. To maintain professionalism in communication you should make all efforts such as including an interpreter if the patient has any language needs or using appropriate communication resources, advocates, or aids for those with intellectual disability. You should always hand over the care of the patient to other colleagues and members of the multi-disciplinary team. You should also ascertain if there are any cultural practices or personal preferences that can impact communication.

Documenting patients' progress and care is an important part of professional communication. A few areas to consider are as follows:

- Ensure your records are accurately recorded
- You may need to enter the date and time of your record
- You should sign off your record to include your name and status
- You should ensure this is countersigned by a Registered Nurse, for example, your practice assessor or supervisor

Another area of professional practice is when you are communicating by email. You should ensure you have an email signature set up so that the receiver of your communication knows who you are and how to contact you. In the case study box below, you will see that Kobi is now a nursing student and has had to set up his email for when he is on placement at the hospital. You will see from his email signature he has provided some information such as his name, designation, the year he started his education, the university he is studying at, the various professionals who are supporting his education, the hospital trust he is attached to, and an email contact.

You may think this all looks simple but often when people receive an email from someone for the first time or someone they don't know, an email signature introduces the individual to that person or group. You can see in some email signatures that individuals who use social media for professional purposes add their details, for example, a LinkedIn profile or Twitter handle.

CASE STUDY

When communicating via email you should remember to always be professional; do not send pictures or images of patients, their results, or medical information unless you have consent to share such sensitive information. If you are ever unsure, always seek support from your practice assessor or practice educator.

This is what your email signature could look like:

Kobi Asante
Nursing student September 2020 Cohort
Insert name of University
BSc Adult Nursing
Cohort Leader: Insert Name
Course Director: Insert Name
Host Trust: Insert Name
Email: Insert email

There are some similarities between spoken and written communication, and one of them is tone. In the same way you will consider the tone, volume, and pitch of your voice when you are talking to someone, you need to be mindful of the tone of your email so that you do not lose professionalism. One such area is using capital or uppercase letters in full words (not acronyms), as this practice is noted as shouting in an email. For example, if you wrote in an email stating, 'PLEASE DO NOT DO THIS AGAIN', the receiver may interpret this as you shouting at them.

Good communication skills (verbal and non-verbal) are essential in nursing and how you approach communication can enhance your professionalism or detract from being professional. In nursing, communicating professionally will help to enhance the way you describe, advocate, and document patients' care and progress.

Team working and mentoring

When caring for a patient you may have to work independently or as part of a team. Working as a team means asking others for help. The people whom you work with are not only Registered Nurses, but they may also come from other healthcare professions such as physiotherapy, occupational therapy, medicine, pharmacy, and social work.

Working together with other allied health professions such as physiotherapists, pharmacists, dieticians, and occupational therapists when caring for a patient is called interprofessional working and demonstrates professionalism as you are acknowledging you cannot work independently at this time and require the support, knowledge, and skills of a team member to provide good and effective patient care. There are also the multi-disciplinary teams which are made up of health and social care professionals that get together to discuss and agree care with the patient and their families. This form of team working or collaborating in care is a two-way process; there will be times when you will also need to offer support to your colleagues. Possessing a collaborative attitude and valuing the support and input of others is a professional behaviour.

Team working can lead to feedback which can be positive or negative, and you will need to develop the professional skill of delivering and receiving feedback. Sharing knowledge and views with team members can build a more professional team and help with bonding and professional growth and development.

During his placement, Kobi's (the case study running throughout this chapter) practice assessor and supervisor discussed with him the importance of having a positive attitude as part of professionalism in nursing.

Use this space to reflect on how you believe positive attitude contributes to professionalism:

_____

_____

_____

_____

_____

_____

Maintain a positive attitude

Your attitude towards patients, their families and carers, and your colleagues can impact how care is delivered, received, and planned. Patients will turn to you for emotional support and your attitude and how you approach situations can impact the way you deliver the emotional support required. Sometimes what you may see as trivial or not requiring much thought or energy may be rated as being of high importance by the patients. Therefore, if you approach support in a laissez-faire manner it can convey to the patient that their concern is not of great importance.

CASE STUDY

Mr Pink was admitted to the ward. He has a pet dog called Bingo and he is very upset as there is no one to look after Bingo. He is visibly worried and keeps asking you what will happen to Bingo. You are not a dog lover and cannot understand why Mr Pink is making such a fuss over a dog and thinks that it's only a dog, and cannot understand why he is so anxious. Your attitude towards not understanding the importance of a pet and how it is part of someone's family can impact the emotional support needed by Mr Pink. The ability to empathise and understand can help to put Mr Pink at ease and relieve his anxiety, which can in turn can help reduce his stress and improve his health.

How might you emotionally support Mr Pink in the case study above?

_____

_____

_____

_____

_____

_____

_____

Your attitude towards your colleagues can impact your working relationships, which can in turn affect the care of the patient. You should try and maintain a positive mental attitude towards work. This involves the words you use to communicate, that is, the way you say things, smiling when you greet someone, offering to help colleagues if you have the time, and offering encouragement to others when and where you can. A positive mental attitude can be demonstrated by respecting others, problem solving together with others, and arriving at new and innovative ideas to work on.

You should also recognise when you need to take a break during the shift and longer in terms of holidays or requested time off. Nursing is a challenging career, and there may be occasions when you do not get the outcome you wanted. It is important when this happens that you seek support through talking to someone or using any services provided by your university or Trust. The Royal College of Nursing's Health Workplace Toolkit (2021) states that 47% of nursing staff felt that they were unable to balance their home and work lives, so it is important to learn to recognise when your mental health is being affected by your work and actions. If you are not in good mental health, you will not be able to perform to the best of your ability and patients and colleagues may interpret this as a negative attitude. This can affect your ability to engage as a team member and impede the way you care.

A positive attitude is integral to being a professional Registered Nurse and if at any time your mental health or any situation impacts your positive attitude then you must seek support. As a student this can be through your personal tutor who offers pastoral care, the Student Services, which offers wellbeing support. Most universities have an entire centre and team dedicated to emotional and physical wellbeing support or the staff support in your trust, and you can also speak to your doctor or general practitioner.

Maintain standards of care

It is a professional responsibility of all Registered Nurses to maintain standards of care; there are several ways as a student you can do this.

- Evidence-based care – you must always deliver evidence-based care. This simply means that the care you administer is grounded in research that is robust and proven to benefit patients and produce desired outcomes. Your nursing course and programme of study should teach you how to search for information on care of different topics. Most library services at university can be accessed online and your librarian or course tutor can provide you with information on how to access online library services. For example, if you need to learn how to treat a patient with sepsis, you can go to the library and search for articles on sepsis treatment. The acute or community healthcare setting where you are working will also have treatment care protocols developed by care teams from national guidance and their own extensive review of the literature. As a nursing student it is a good idea to start by looking at what a person's treatment plan is and have a discussion with your practice assessor or supervisor on how these plans constitute evidence-based care. You should also ensure that the advice you give any patient is evidence based. For example, if the patient is living with diabetes, giving information on types of medication and dietary and lifestyle management should be evidence based.

- Following the Code – in the UK the Nursing and Midwifery Council is the regulatory body for Registered Nurses, Midwives, Health Visitors and Nursing Associates. The NMC has developed the Code, which helps Registered Nurses to stay professional; it presents the standards that Registered Nurses, Midwives, Health Visitors, and Nursing Associates must adhere to and uphold to be able to practise in the UK.

All students who aspire to register as a practitioner with the NMC are expected to uphold the Code and be knowledgeable of its content. The NMC also provides guidance on other areas that help you to stay professional and practise professionally and effectively; for example, there is guidance on how to maintain professionalism online, particularly regarding social media (NMC 2022a).

- Joining a Nursing Association or Nursing Union – belonging to a professional organisation such as an association or union can help you to develop a professional image and professional practice. The nursing association or union has the potential to keep you informed about new developments and changes in the nursing field and provide you with a different perspective. This is done through their membership newsletter, and some have monthly magazines you can access as a member. Such organisations can provide educational support and networking opportunities with wider members through forum memberships and can advise on career pathways, including job application support and interview techniques. There is also the peer recognition of being part of an organisation as well as the identity as an affiliated member of a professional group. The Chief Nursing Officer for England, Ruth May, has created a budget to help develop nursing associations from different countries working in England; for example, there is the Caribbean Nursing and Midwifery Association, Filipino Nurse Association, British Indian Nurse Association, British Sikh Association, and the Kenyan Nursing Association, amongst others. There is also a CNO BME Strategic Advisory Group that supports ethnic minority Registered Nurses and advises the CNO of England.

- Be accountable and honest – professionalism is linked to your integrity, honesty, and transparency. Taking personal responsibility for your practice including being accountable for any mistakes you may have made is good practice. As a student you will need to learn to document the care you have delivered as well as the decisions you have made. Documentation in nursing is important; what you have written makes you accountable for your practice and also acts as a form of communication with other Registered Nurses and members of the multi-disciplinary team. You may administer medication under supervision, and you should document this in the patient's notes or you may have to countersign in the medical administration record, commonly called the drug chart. It's also important to understand that you have a duty of candour, which means as a Registered Nurse or nursing student you should be open and transparent in your actions. For example, if a patient was given the incorrect drug or dosage, the Registered Nurse administering the medication should disclose and discuss this with the patient. Honesty is a professional trait, and you should be honest and transparent about all care you provide to the patient. When you discuss with a patient or their family that you have made an error this practice is called candour and the NMC (2022b) and GMC (General Medical Council) have produced a joint statement called the professional duty of candour.

Duty of candour

You make sure that patient and public safety is not affected. You work within the limits of your competence, exercising your professional 'duty of candour' and raising concerns immediately whenever you come across situations that put patients or public safety at risk. You take necessary action to deal with any concerns where appropriate

The Code

As a Registered Nurse, Midwife, Health Visitor or Nursing Associate you must uphold the professional standards set out by the NMC. These professional standards are called the Code and, like other registered professionals, these have been developed to ensure clear regulatory principles outlining what is required of those registered individuals.

As you progress through your nursing education you will see that the Code is the foundation on which all Registered Nurses, Midwives, health Visitors and Nursing Associates practice. The Code acts as a guide that directs and provides accountability tools for registrants on their responsibilities as registered healthcare professionals. It can also be used as a tool to support reflection and decision making, as well as their learning and development, and for revalidation.

The NMC professional Code became effective in March 2015 following a consultation period whereby the previous Code of Conduct (2008) was updated to reflect modern nursing practice. The current Code published in 2018 was amended to include the new role of nursing associates in England. As we have already discussed, the NMC's Code contains the professional standards that Registered Nurses, Midwives, health Visitors and Nursing Associates must uphold. Any individual who is on the NMC register must act in line with the Code, whether they are providing direct care to individuals, groups, or communities. This would also include those who are working in other roles such as leadership, education, or research. The Code can be applied in a range of different practice settings, and they are not negotiable or discretionary.

As you can see below, The Code contains several statements and together they signify what good practice looks like. It ensures that the interests of patients and service users are put first, ensuring that an individual's practice is safe and effective as well as promoting trust through professionalism.

Reading and understanding the Code is an integral part of practising as a Registered Nurse, Midwife, Health Visitor or Nursing Associate in the UK and allows those practising to deliver high-quality care and also guides registrants on the revalidation process. Revalidation is a process you will have to engage with after you qualify; it occurs every 3 years and helps you to maintain your registration. Essentially the Code guides your conduct and is a summary of the profession; it also sets out rules of behaviour and professionalism that Registered Nurses including students must follow while reflecting the personal accountability and personal responsibility that a registrant must convey within their role.

During your practice as a nursing student, you will hear conversations about the Nursing and Midwifery Council. It is important that you understand how the Council operates and their role in your profession. The Nursing and Midwifery Council (NMC) is the regulatory body that oversees the practice of all Registered Nurses, Midwives, health Visitors and Nursing Associates. As an organisation they set standards for practice, hold a register, quality-assure education, and investigate complaints made against any practitioner that is on the register (NMC 2018).

The NMC regulates almost 745,000 nursing and midwifery professionals. Their core role is to promote high standards of education and professional standards for Registered Nurses, Midwives,Health Visitors and Nursing Associates across the UK while also maintaining the register of those who can practise. The NMC are also responsible for investigating complaints that are made against Registered Nurses, Midwives, Health Visitors and Nursing Associates (NMC 2022c). While they believe that all professionals should be given a chance to address concerns that are raised in practice, they can act when required and place conditions on those eligible to practise or in more serious cases stop individuals from being able to practise in the UK.

Four Principles of Professionalism (NMC)

The NMC has four main principles: prioritise people, practise effectively, preserve safety, and promote trust and professionalism. We outline these for you below.

NMC

THE CODE SAYS

Prioritise People

To acheive this you must:

1. Treat people as individuals and uphold their dignity
2. Listen to people and respond to their preferences and concerns
3. Make sure that people's physical, social and psychological needs are assessed and responded to
4. Act in the best interests of people at all times
5. Respect people's right to privacy and confidentiality

Practise Effectively

To acheive this you must:

6. Always practise in line with the best available evidence
7. Communicate early
8. Work co-operatively
9. Share your skills, knowledge and experience for the benefit of people receiving care and your colleagues
10. Keep clear and accurate records relevant to your practice
11. Be accountable for your decisions to delegate tasks and duties to other people
12. Have in place an indemnity arrangement which provides appropriate cover for any practice you take on as a nurse, midwife or nursing associate in the United Kingdom

Preserve Safety

To acheive this you must:

13. Recognise and work within the limits of your competence
14. Be open and candid with all service users about all aspects of care and treatment, including when any mistakes or harm have taken place
15. Always offer help if an emergency arises in your practice setting or anywhere else
16. Act without delay if you believe that there is a risk to patient safety or public protection
17. Raise concerns immediately if you believe a person is vulnerable or at risk and needs extra support and protection

18. Advise on, prescribe, supply, dispense or administer medicines within the limits of your training and competence, the law, our guidance and other relevant policies, guidance and regulations
19. Be aware of, and reduce as far as possible, any potential for harm associated with your practice

Promote Professionalism and Trust

To acheive this you must:

20. Uphold the reputation of your profession at all times
21. Uphold your position as a Registered Nurse, Midwife or Nursing Associate
22. Fulfil all registration requirements
23. Cooperate with all investigations and audits
24. Respond to any complaints made against you professionally
25. Provide leadership to make sure people's wellbeing is protected and to improve their experiences of the health and care system

While the statements above outline the expectations of a Registered Nurse, Midwife, Health Visitor or Nursing Associate, the Code also outlines how they expect an individual on the register to achieve the principles.

Prioritise people

You must put the interests of people using or needing nursing or midwifery services first. You should make their care and safety the main concern and ensure that their dignity is preserved, and their needs are recognised, assessed, and responded to. You will also need to make sure that those receiving care are treated with respect, that their rights are upheld, and that any discriminatory attitudes and behaviours towards those receiving care are challenged.

One of the fundamentals of nursing and midwifery clinical practice is prioritising patients. Ensuring that those who receive care are treated with respect and have their dignity maintained is a key priority. It is important to listen to patients and be responsive to their preferences and concerns. It would be expected that wherever this level of care was not provided by a Registered Nurse, Midwife, Health Visitor or Nursing Associate, this would be appropriately escalated and, where required, reported to the NMC.

NMC

THE CODE SAYS

1. **Treat people as individuals and uphold their dignity**
   To achieve this, you must:
   1.1. treat people with kindness, respect and compassion
   1.2. make sure you deliver the fundamentals of care effectively
   1.3. avoid making assumptions and recognise diversity and individual choice
   1.4. make sure that any treatment, assistance or care for which you are responsible is delivered without undue delay
   1.5. respect and uphold people's human rights

2. **Listen to people and respond to their preferences and concerns**
   To achieve this, you must:
   2.1. work in partnership with people to make sure you deliver care effectively
   2.2. recognise and respect the contribution that people can make to their own health and wellbeing
   2.3. encourage and empower people to share in decisions about their own treatment and care
   2.4. respect the level to which people receiving care want to be involved in decisions about their own health, wellbeing and care
   2.5. respect, support and document a person's right to accept or refuse care and treatment
   2.6. recognise when people are anxious or in distress and respond compassionately and politely

3. **Make sure that people's physical, social and psychological needs are assessed and responded to**
   To achieve this, you must:
   3.1. pay special attention to promoting wellbeing, preventing ill health and meeting the changing health and care needs of people during all life stages
   3.2. recognise and respond compassionately to the needs of those who are in the last few days and hours of life

3.3. act in partnership with those receiving care, helping them to access relevant health and social care, information and support when they need it

3.4. act as an advocate for the vulnerable, challenging poor practice and discriminatory attitudes and behaviour relating to their care

4. **Act in the best interest of people at all times**

4.1. balance the need to act in the best interest of people at all times with the requirement to respect a person's right to accept or refuse treatment

4.2. make sure that you get properly informed consent and document it before carrying out any action

4.3. keep to all relevant laws about mental capacity that apply in the country in which you are practising, and make sure that the rights and best interests of those who lack capacity are still at the centre of the decision-making process

4.4. tell colleagues, your manager and the person receiving care if you have a conscientious objection to a particular procedure and arrange for a suitably qualified colleague to take over responsibility for that person's care

5. **Respect people's right to privacy and confidentiality**

To achieve this, you must:

5.1. respect a person's right to privacy in all aspects of their care

5.2. make sure that people are informed about how and why information is used and shared by those who will be providing care

5.3. respect that a person's right to privacy and confidentiality continues after they have died

5.4. share necessary information with other health and care professionals and agencies only when the interest of patient safety and public protection override the need for confidentiality

5.5. share with people, their families, and their carers, as far as the law allows, the information they want or need to know about their health, care and ongoing treatment sensitively and in a way they can understand

Practise effectively

You must assess the needs of patients and deliver or advise on treatment or give help (including both preventative or rehabilitative care) without too much of a delay. You are also expected to provide treatment to the best of your abilities based on the best available evidence. You must communicate effectively, ensuring that you keep clear and accurate records and share skills, knowledge, and experience where appropriate. As a Registered Nurse, Midwife, Health Visitor or Nursing Associate you should reflect on practice and act on any feedback that you receive to improve your practice.

To practise effectively you should keep your skills up to date and continually expand on your knowledge within your chosen field. One of the ways in which this can be completed is through attending a training session and continuing professional development; this will help you maintain up-to-date knowledge and deliver safe and effective practice. When practising effectively, it is also important to keep up to date with national guidelines such as those published by the National Institute for Health and Care Excellence (NICE) but also discipline-specific bodies such as the British Thoracic Society (BTS) and SIGN in Scotland.

NMC

THE CODE SAYS

6. **Always practise in line with the best available evidence**
   To achieve this, you must:
   6.1. make sure that any information or advice given is evidence-based including information relating to using any health and care products or services
   6.2. maintain the knowledge and skills you need for safe and effective practice

7. **Communicate clearly**
   To achieve this, you must:
   7.1. use terms that people in your care, colleagues and the public can understand
   7.2. take reasonable steps to meet people's language and communication needs, providing, wherever possible, assistance to those who need help to communicate their own or other people's needs

7.3. use a range of verbal and non-verbal communication methods, and consider cultural sensitivities, to better understand and respond to people's personal and health needs

7.4. check people's understanding from time to time to keep misunderstanding or mistakes to a minimum

7.5. be able to communicate clearly and effectively in English

8. **Work co-operatively**

To achieve this, you must:

8.1. respect the skills, expertise and contributions of your colleagues, referring matters to them when appropriate

8.2. maintain effective communication with colleagues

8.3. keep colleagues informed when you are sharing the care of individuals with other health and care professionals and staff

8.4. work with colleagues to evaluate the quality of your work and that of the team

8.5. work with colleagues to preserve the safety of those receiving care

8.6. share information to identify and reduce risk

8.7. be supportive of colleagues who are encountering health or performance problems. However, this support must never compromise or be at the expense of patient or public safety

9. **Share your skills, knowledge and experience for the benefit of people receiving care and your colleagues**

To achieve this, you must:

9.1. provide honest, accurate and constructive feedback to colleagues

9.2. gather and reflect on feedback from a variety of sources, using it to improve your practice and performance

9.3. deal with differences of professional opinion with colleagues by discussion and informed debate, respecting their views and opinions and behaving in a professional way at all times

9.4. support students and colleagues learning to help them develop their professional competence and confidence

10. **Keep clear and accurate records relevant to your practice**

This applies to the records that are relevant to your scope of practice. It includes but is not limited to patient records.

Continued

To a chieve this, you must:

10.1. complete records at the time or as soon as possible after an event, recording if the notes are written some time after the event

10.2. identify any risks or problems that have arisen and the steps taken to deal with them, so that colleagues who use the records have all the information they need

10.3. complete records accurately and without any falsification, taking immediate and appropriate action if you become aware that someone has not kept to these requirements

10.4. attribute any entries you make in any paper or electronic records to yourself, making sure they are clearly written, dated and timed, and do not include unnecessary abbreviations, jargon or speculation

10.5. take all steps to make sure that records are kept securely

10.6. collect, treat and store all data and research findings appropriately

11. **Be accountable for your decisions to delegate tasks and duties to other people**
To achieve this you must

11.1. only delegate tasks and duties that are within the other person's scope of competence, making sure that they fully understand your instructions

11.2. make sure that everyone you delegate tasks to is adequately supervised and supported so they can provide safe and compassionate care

11.3. confirm that the outcome of any task you have delegated to someone else meets the required standard

12. **Have in place an indemnity arrangement which provides appropriate cover for any practice you take on as a nurse, midwife or nursing associate in the United Kingdom**
To achieve this, you must:

12.1. make sure that you have an appropriate indemnity arrangement in place relevant to your scope of practice.

Preserve safety

As a Registered Nurse, Midwife, Health Visitor or Nursing Associate you must make sure that patient and public safety is not affected and that you work within your limits of competence. You must also exercise your professional 'duty of candour' and raise concerns immediately whenever you come across a situation that puts patients or public safety at risk. You are also expected to take the necessary action to deal with any concerns where appropriate.

An essential part of persevering safety in practice is to be open and honest when mistakes are made regarding a patient's care, particularly when this has the potential to cause harm. It is important that you undertake the necessary training to preserve safety within your chosen speciality and continue to undertake training, ensuring you are provided with the most up-to-date evidence and guidance. An example of this would be working in a critical care setting, whereby you would need to undertake further education and competencies to practise autonomously. As a Registered Nurse, Midwife, Health Visitor or Nursing Associate, you should follow not only the NMC code of conduct regarding professional behaviour but also the local policies and procedures, to reduce the risk of any potential harm associated with your practice.

NMC

THE CODE SAYS

13. **Recognise and work within the limits of your competence**
    To achieve this, you must:
    13.1. accurately identify, observe and assess signs of normal or worsening physical and mental health in the person receiving care
    13.2. make a timely referral to another practitioner when any action, care or treatment is required
    13.3. ask for help from a suitably qualified and experienced professional to carry out any action or procedure that is beyond the limits of your competence
    13.4. take account of your own personal safety as well as the safety of people in your care
    13.5. complete the necessary training before carrying out a new role

Continued

14. **Be open and candid with all service users about all aspects of care and treatment, including when any mistakes or harm have taken place**

To achieve this, you must:

14.1. act immediately to put right the situation if someone has suffered actual harm for any reason or an incident has happened which had the potential for harm

14.2. explain fully and promptly what has happened, including the likely effects, and apologise to the person affected and, where appropriate, their advocate, family or carers

14.3. document all these events formally and take further action (escalate) if appropriate so they can be dealt with quickly

15. **Always offer help if an emergency arises in your practice setting or anywhere else**

To achieve this, you must:

15.1. only act in an emergency within the limits of your knowledge and competence

15.2. arrange, wherever possible, for emergency care to be accessed and provided promptly

15.3. take account of your own safety, the safety of others and the availability of other options for providing care

16. **Act without delay if you believe that there is a risk to patient safety or public protection**

To achieve this, you must:

16.1. raise and, if necessary, escalate any concerns you may have about patient or public safety, or the level of care people are receiving in your workplace or any other health and care setting and use the channels available to you in line with our guidance and your local working practices

16.2. raise your concerns immediately if you are being asked to practise beyond your role, experience and training

16.3. tell someone in authority at the first reasonable opportunity if you experience problems that may prevent you working within The Code or other national standards, taking prompt action to tackle the causes of concern if you can

16.4. acknowledge and act on all concerns raised to you, investigating, escalating or dealing with those concerns where it is appropriate for you to do so

16.5. not obstruct, intimidate, victimise or in any way hinder a colleague, member of staff, person you care for or member of the public who wants to raise a concern

16.6. protect anyone you have management responsibility for from any harm, detriment, victimisation or unwarranted treatment after a concern is raised

17. Raise concerns immediately if you believe a person is vulnerable or at risk and needs extra support and protection
To achieve this, you must:

17.1. take all reasonable steps to protect people who are vulnerable or at risk of harm, neglect or abuse

17.2. share information if you believe someone may be at risk of harm, in line with the laws relating to the disclosure of information

17.3. have knowledge of and keep to the relevant laws and policies about protecting and caring for vulnerable people

18. Advise on, prescribe, supply, dispense or administer medicines within the limits of your training and competence, the law, our guidance and other relevant policies, guidance and regulations
To achieve this, you must:

18.1. prescribe, advise on, or provide medicines or treatment, including repeat prescriptions (only if you are suitably qualified) if you have enough knowledge of that persons health and are satisfied that the medicines or treatment serve that persons health needs

18.2. keep to appropriate guidelines when giving advice on using controlled drugs and recording the prescribing, supply, dispensing or administration of controlled drugs

18.3. make sure that the care or treatment you advise on, prescribe, supply, dispense or administer for each person is compatible with any other care or treatment they are receiving, including (where possible) over-the-counter medicines

18.4. take all steps to keep medicines stored securely

18.5. wherever possible, avoid prescribing for yourself or for anyone with whom you have a close personal relationship

Continued

19. **Be aware of, and reduce as far as possible any potential for harm associated with your practice**
To achieve this you must:
19.1. take measures to reduce as far as possible, the likelihood of mistakes, near misses, harm and the effect of harm if it takes place
19.2. take account of current evidence, knowledge and developments in reducing mistakes and the effect of them and the impact of human factors and system failures
19.3. keep to and promote the recommended practice in relation to controlling and preventing infection
19.4. take all reasonable personal precautions necessary to avoid any potential health risks to colleagues, people receiving care and the public

Prescribing is not within the scope of practice for everyone on the NMC's register. Nursing associates do not prescribe, but they may supply, dispense and administer medicines. Registered Nurses and Midwives who have successfully completed a further qualification in prescribing and have recorded it on the NMC's register are the only people that than can prescribe.

Promote professionalism and trust

As a Registered Nurse, Midwife, Health Visitor or Nursing Associate you must uphold the reputation of your profession at all times. You need to display a personal commitment to the standards of practice and behaviours that are set out by the Code, as well as being a model of integrity and leadership that others aspire to. This should lead to trust and confidence in the professions from patients, people receiving care, other health and care professionals, and the public.

While the Code exists to demonstrate the professional behaviours and illustrate good practice of a Registered Nurse, Midwife, Health Visitor or

Nursing Associate, it is important to note that this does not only apply when practising and is applied to everything that you do. For example, the NMC could investigate a post or image on a personal social media account that brought the profession into disrepute. As a Registered Nurse, Midwife, Health Visitor or Nursing Associate, you should behave in a way that inspires public trust and confidence, ensuring that a trusting relationship has been developed with patients, which is essential to their care.

NMC

THE CODE SAYS

20. Uphold the reputation of your profession at all times
To achieve this, you must:
20.1. keep to and uphold the standards and values set out in the Code
20.2. act with honesty and integrity at all times, treating people fairly and without discrimination, bullying or harassment
20.3. be aware at all times of how your behaviour can affect and influence the behaviour of other people
20.4. keep to the laws of the country in which you are practising
20.5. treat people in a way that does not take advantage of their vulnerability or cause them upset or distress
20.6. stay objective and have clear professional boundaries at all times with people in your care (including those who have been in your care in the past), their families and carers
20.7. make sure you do not express your personal beliefs (including political, religious or moral beliefs) to people in an inappropriate way
20.8. act as a role model of professional behaviour for students and newly qualified nurses, midwives and nursing associates to aspire to
20.9. maintain the level of health you need to carry out your professional role
20.10. use all forms of spoken, written and digital communication (including social media and networking sites) responsibly, respecting the right to privacy of others at all times

Continued

21. **Uphold your position as a registered nurse, midwife or nursing associate**

To achieve this, you must:

21.1. refuse all but the most trivial gifts, favours or hospitality as accepting them could be interpreted as an attempt to gain preferential treatment

21.2. never ask for or accept loans from anyone in your care or anyone close to them

21.3. act with honesty and integrity in any financial dealings you have with everyone you have professional relationship with, including people in your care

21.4. make sure that any advertisement, publications or published material you produce or have produced for your professional services are accurate, responsible, ethical, do not mislead or exploit vulnerabilities and accurately reflect your relevant skills, experience and qualifications

21.5. never use your status as a registered professional to promote causes that are not related to health

21.6. cooperate with the media only when it is appropriate to do so, and then always protecting the confidentiality and dignity of people receiving treatment or care

22. **Fulfil all registration requirements**

To achieve this, you must:

22.1. keep to any reasonable requests so we can oversee the registration process

22.2. keep to your prescribed hours of practice and carry out continuing professional development activities

22.3. keep your knowledge and skills up to date, taking part in appropriate and regular learning and professional development activities that aim to maintain and develop your competence and improve your performance

23. **Cooperate with all investigations and audits**

This includes investigation or audits either against you or relating to others, whether individuals or organisations. It also includes cooperating with requests to act as a witness in any hearing that forms part of an investigation, even after you have left the register.

To achieve this, you must:

23.1. cooperate with any audits of training records, registration records or other relevant audits that we may want to carry out to make sure you are still fit to practise

23.2. tell both us and any employers as soon as you can about any caution or charge against you, or if you have received a conditional discharge in relation to, or have been found guilty of, a criminal offence (other than a protected caution or conviction)

23.3. tell us and employers you work for if you have had your practice restricted or had any other conditions imposed on you by us or any other relevant body

23.4. tell us and your employers at the first reasonable opportunity if you are or have been disciplined by any regulatory or licensing organisation, including those who operate outside of the professional health and care environment

23.5. give your NMC Pin when any reasonable request for it is made

24. **Respond to any complaints made against you professionally**
   To achieve this, you must:

24.1. never allow someone's complaint to affect the care that is provided to them

24.2. use all complaints as a form of feedback and an opportunity for reflection and learning to improve practice

25. **Provide leadership to make sure people wellbeing is protected and to improve their experiences of the health and care system**
   To achieve this you must:

25.1. identify priorities, manage time, staff and resources effectively and deal with risk to make sure that the quality of care or service you deliver is maintained and improved, putting the needs of those receiving care and services first

25.2. support any staff you may be responsible for to follow the Code at all times. They must have the knowledge, skills and competence for safe practice; and understand how to raise any concerns linked to any circumstances where the Code has, or could be, broken

FITNESS TO PRACTISE

The core role of the NMC is to regulate the practice of Registered Nurses, Midwives, health Visitors and Nursing Associates within the UK. One of the ways in which this can be done is by investigating concerns that have been raised. These concerns can be raised by anyone, for example, another health professional, a patient or their family, a member of the public, or an employer. The NMC acts to protect the public. It is important to note that while this is one of the core roles of the NMC, less than 1% of registrants are investigated each year. The aim of this process is not to punish individuals but to ensure that all registrants meet the set standards and practice safely. When investigating whether a registrant is 'fit to practise', the Code is used to assess whether an individual has fallen below the expected standard. The overall process allows the NMC to understand whether an individual is a risk to the public and can put processes in place to promote learning and prevent such issues from arising again (NMC 2018).

The NMC takes any concern that has been raised very seriously, and there are several different steps in the process of deciding whether a concern should be investigated.

Fitness to Practise for nursing students and student midwives

In 2009 all universities with a nursing faculty referred to as approved education institutions (AEI) were required to set up their own fitness to practise committee to consider any pre-registration nursing student's fitness to practise regarding health and character. A local fitness to practise panel exists to consider health or character issues and to protect the public.

Local fitness to practise panels should only be used if a student's health or disability is likely to compromise or has compromised their ability to meet the required competencies and practise safely.

If necessary, a local fitness to practise panel will meet to decide about a student's suitability to remain on the programme. This would apply if your attitude or behaviour is such that it calls into question your good character.

Health

You must disclose to your AEI any health conditions and/or disability when you apply to study to be a Registered Nurse, Midwife, Health Visitor or Nursing Associate which could affect your ability to practise safely and effectively.

Your AEI will provide a supporting declaration for you in relation to your health when you come to register with the NMC. Usually, the director or leader of your nursing programme will get you to fill in a health declaration annually.

When the NMC assesses your health condition and/or disability, they will check whether you have disclosed your health condition and/or disability to your educational institution.

You should speak to your educational institution if you have any questions about what you need to declare to them.

Character

You will be required to tell your education institution of any police charges, cautions, convictions, or conditional discharges when you apply to study to be a Registered Nurse, Midwife, Health Visitor or Nursing Associate.

If you're charged with a criminal offence or receive a caution, conviction, or conditional discharge while you are studying, you must tell your education institution. Your education institution will then investigate to decide if it calls into question whether you are of good character to remain on the course.

If you remain on the course, your educational institution will provide a supporting declaration for you in relation to your character when you come to register with the NMC. You must also declare the charge, caution, conviction, or conditional discharge to the NMC when applying to join the register, unless it is protected.

When the NMC assesses your character, they will check whether you have disclosed the police charge, caution, conviction, or conditional discharge to your education institution.

You should speak to your educational institution if you have any questions about what you need to declare to them.

Fitness to Practise and racial discrimination

Racism exists in the nursing profession (Moorley et al. 2020), and the current fitness to practise system in the NMC acknowledges this discrimination exists. A research work led by Professor West at the University of Greenwich 2017 found the following.

- The progress and outcomes of Black and Minority Ethnic (BME) Registered Nurses and Midwives through the Fitness to Practise (FtP) process of the Nursing and Midwifery Council (NMC) has shown that ethnicity is related to the risk of referral to the NMC. Black Registered Nurses and Midwives as well as those of Unknown ethnicity are disproportionately represented in the population of referrals to the NMC. Having qualified in Africa, as opposed to other continents, is also a risk factor for referral. It is important to note, however, that ethnicity is known for only 60% of referrals. In the absence of more complete data on ethnicity, it cannot yet be concluded with certainty that some ethnic groups run a greater risk of referral.
- BME males are more likely to be referred to the NMC than are White male Registered Nurses and Midwives who are under-represented in referrals.
- There are many sources of referral to the NMC but the most common are employers and members of the public. BME Registered Nurses and Midwives are disproportionately represented in referrals by employers, whereas White Registered Nurses and Midwives are disproportionately represented in referrals by members of the public. Source of referral is extremely consequential in terms of progress and outcomes of the FtP process.
- Ethnicity is also related to progression through the FtP process. Cases brought against Registered Nurses and Midwives of White, Other, or Unknown ethnicities are more likely to be closed at screening than are cases brought against Asian or Black Registered

Nurses and Midwives whose cases are more likely to be closed at the investigation stage.

- Region of training is also related to progression through the FtP process. Having trained outside the UK increases the likelihood of the case going to investigation and having trained in Asia or Africa increases the risk of the case going to adjudication.
- Referrals by employers in which BME Registered Nurses and Midwives are over-represented are unlikely to be closed at screening and most likely to be closed at investigation. A significant number of employer referrals go on to adjudication, which contributes to the increased likelihood of BME Registered Nurses and Midwives going all the way to the last stage of the FtP process. (NMC 2022d)

CASE STUDY

The case of the Registered Nurse Melanie Hayes is one example of the type of racism Registered Nurses experience. Hayes was a Registered Nurse who verbally abused colleagues at work, making racist statements, and her colleagues made a formal complaint to the hospital that employed her and she was referred to the NMC. In the initial hearing the actions of the Registered Nurse in question were deemed as not causing much harm to those involved, and a petition was then raised by Registered Nurses and the NMC had to re-open and re-investigate the case. This case was also one of learning for the NMC on how they assess cases of racism. The NMC has published their report: *Looking back, learning lessons and improving Discrimination in health and care: learning from a recent fitness to practise case* (NMC 2022e)

As a nursing student you will need to learn how to deal with and manage racism in practice. You may witness racism against colleagues or patients and you will need to use your communication skills and your employer's or University's policies on discrimination.

NMC

THE CODE SAYS

You put the interests of people using or needing nursing or midwifery services first. You make their care and safety your main concern and make sure that their dignity is preserved and their needs are recognised, assessed and responded to. You make sure that those receiving care are treated with respect, that their rights are upheld and that any discriminatory attitudes and behaviours towards those receiving care are challenged.

CONCLUSION

In this chapter we have explored what professionalism as a student looks like and how you can develop into a professional Registered Nurse and maintain a professional outlook and practice. We have provided you with case studies of real-life nursing student experiences and how they act out in the clinical practice setting. This chapter also gives you some useful tips on how to become and stay professional as a Registered Nurse. We introduced you to the NMC and some of the key principles that guide your practice; this includes The Code, guidelines for using social media, being honest and transparent through the duty of candour, and understanding discrimination such as racism. This chapter aims to help you to understand diversity and being professional when working with diverse patient and staff groups. As a nursing student it is very important that you understand how the NMC operates and how The Code provides guidance for our professional practice.

Having read the chapter on professionalism please add your thoughts and reflections

_____

_____

_____

_____

_____

_____

_____

_____

_____

_____

_____

_____

_____

_____

_____

_____

_____

_____

_____

_____

_____

REFERENCES

Capparelli, J.L. (2005). Nursing Nuns: A history of caring – And changing the course of health care. *The American Journal of Nursing*, *105*(8), p. 72H.

Moorley, C., Darbyshire, P., Serrant, L., Mohamed, J., Ali, P. and De Souza, R. (2020). Dismantling structural racism: Nursing must not be caught on the wrong side of history. *Journal of Advanced Nursing*, *76*(10), pp. 2450–2453.

Moorly, C. and Puthenpurakal, A. (2019). Professional skills for adult ursing. In Moorley C., ed. Introductions to Nursing for First Year Students. p. 72. Available at https://uk.sagepub.com/en-gb/eur/introduction-to-nursing-for-first-year-students/book258583

Nursing and Midwifery Council. (2017). Enabling professionalism in nursing and midwifery practice. London: Nursing and Midwifery Council. Available at https://www.nmc.org.uk/globalassets/sitedocuments/other-publications/enabling-professionalism.pdf

Nursing and Midwifery Council. (2018). *The Code: Professional Standards of Practice and Behaviour for Nurses, Midwives and Nursing Associates*. London: Nursing & Midwifery Council.

Nursing and Midwifery Council. (2022a). Guidance on using social media responsibly. Available at https://www.nmc.org.uk/globalassets/sitedocuments/nmc-publications/social-media-guidance.pdf

Nursing and Midwifery Council. (2022b). The professional duty of candour. Available at https://www.nmc.org.uk/standards/guidance/the-professional-duty-of-candour/read-the-professional-duty-of-candour/

Nursing and Midwifery Council. (2022c). Home page. Available at https://www.nmc.org.uk/

Nursing and Midwifery Council. (2022d). Fitness to practise report. Available at https://www.nmc.org.uk/globalassets/sitedocuments/other-publications/bme-nurses—midwives-ftp-research-report.pdf

Nursing and Midwifery Council. (2022e). Looking back, learning lessons and improving Discrimination in health and care: Learning from a recent fitness to practise case.

Available at https://www.nmc.org.uk/globalassets/sitedocuments/ftp/hayes-report.pdf

Royal College of Nursing. (2021). Healthy workplace toolkit. Available at https://www.rcn.org.uk/Professional-Development/publications/healthy-workplace-toolkit-uk-pub-009-734

West, E., Nayar, S., Taskila, T. and Al-Haboubi, M. (2017). *The Progress and Outcomes of Black and Minority Ethnic (BME) Nurses and Midwives through the Nursing and Midwifery Council's Fitness to Practise Process*. London: University of Greenwich.

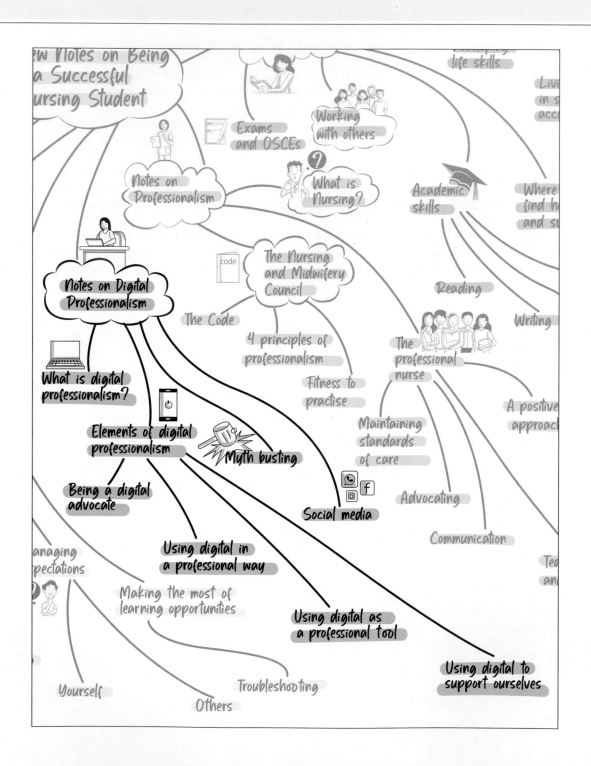

NOTES ON DIGITAL PROFESSIONALISM

Teresa Chinn (She/Her)   ■   Joy O'Gorman (He/Him)

INTRODUCTION

Digital professionalism is a concept that nursing students need to grasp early in their nursing journey. Being digital in nursing is integral to being part of a global profession; the way we portray ourselves online; the way we behave online; the way we use digital with, and for, the people we care for; and how we use digital to support ourselves and our colleagues, all play an important part of nursing.

With growing backlogs and pressures, digital platforms have become an important ally in health and care delivery services (NHSx 2022; World Health Organization [WHO] 2021). Furthermore, the Covid-19 pandemic created a rapid shift to online patient consultations, virtual community wards, simulated learning, and technology-enhanced placements. Therefore, it is important we learn how to be digitally professional as an individual registrant and as part of the wider multidisciplinary team.

But what do we mean by the term digital professionalism? What does it look like in practice? What are the important things that nursing students need to get to grips with? This chapter aims to explore all of these things and provide a taster of the concept of digital professionalism in nursing.

WHAT IS DIGITAL PROFESSIONALISM?

Before we can explore digital professionalism it's important to first explain what is meant by digital. There are lots of definitions that seek to define 'digital' as binary data, for example, or computerised driven technology. Broader concepts view digital as less of a 'thing' but as a cultural change and a new way of engaging with others (McKinsey & Company 2015). In terms of health, digital transformations are changing the way in which we work and relate to service users and others.

The Personalised HealthCare 2020 states that 'better use of data and technology has the power to improve health, transforming the quality and reducing the cost of health and care services' (Gov.UK 2014). The World Health Organization's digital strategy for global health 2020–2025 defines digital health as an umbrella term comprising a broad range of technologies (2021). A key goal of NHS England & Improvement is to accelerate the digital transformation of the NHS, drawing on fast-paced changes made during the pandemic (NHSx 2022). Furthermore, NHS England's (2021) Chief Nursing Officer current strategic plan for research includes a call for digitally enabled nurse-led research.

Therefore, embracing digital is an important foundation for any current and future Registered Nurses as healthcare services respond to evolving demands and growth.

Professionalism

Professionalism is woven throughout the Nursing and Midwifery Council (NMC) Code (NMC 2018) and has its very own section, 'Promote professionalism and trust,' which explores the expectations of the NMC in regard to Registered Nurses and professionalism.

NMC

THE CODE SAYS

'You uphold the reputation of your profession at all times. You should display a personal commitment to the standards of practice and behaviour set out in the Code. You should be a model of integrity and leadership for others to aspire to. This should lead to trust and confidence in the profession from patients, people receiving care, other health and care professionals and the public'

However, there is only one section of the code that specifically mentions digital – section 20.10. This doesn't mean to say that this is the only part of the NMC Code that is relevant, though; the entire NMC Code applies to all Registered Nurses regardless of settings or context and this includes digital settings and contexts.

NMC

THE CODE SAYS

20.10   Use all forms of spoken, written and digital communication (including social media and networking sites) responsibly, respecting the right to privacy of others at all times

The NMC code doesn't explore or define the concept of digital professionalism; it simply adheres to the mandate that Registered Nurses should remain professional and therefore digitally professional. A further document from the NMC, 'Enabling professionalism in nursing and midwifery practice' (NMC 2017), explores the concept of professionalism in greater depth. 'Professionalism is characterised by the autonomous evidence-based decision making by members of an occupation who share the same values and education. Professionalism in nursing and midwifery is realised through purposeful relationships and underpinned by environments that facilitate professional practice. Professional nurses and midwives demonstrate and embrace accountability for their actions'. The NMC expand on this definition by identifying four main areas of professionalism:

- Being accountable (Practise effectively)
- Being a leader (Promote professionalism and trust)
- Being an advocate (Prioritise people)
- Being competent (Preserve safety)

The NMC code and 'Enabling professionalism in nursing and midwifery practice' work together to set the expectation for digital professionalism in nursing. In essence, digital professionalism in nursing is about being competent and applying all aspects of the NMC code to digital spaces whilst being accountable, leading, and advocating. It's important to remember that digital professionalism applies to all aspects of nursing in digital spaces such as social media, e-mail, apps, use of digital technology, and data.

TWEET

@PhilBallRN

'Being a professional (not attempting to define a professional) at all times, when communicating - adding digital doesn't alter the need for a that approach, just a shift in the nature of the tools we have at our disposal?'

TWEET

@CharlotteNHSRN

'Digital capabilities and competence, which includes a progressive attitude towards technology and innovation and its potential to improve our services and healthcare care outcomes. To achieve this, we need to develop our digital literacy amongst the healthcare workforce'

The elements of digital professionalism

Digital professionalism can seem like an abstract concept that can be confusing when applied to practical situations. It's hard to understand how to be competent or a leader in digital spaces; therefore it is not merely enough to define digital professionalism.

In order to be digitally professional as a nursing student the idea needs to be broken down into its practical elements. Chinn (2019) suggests that the practical application of digital professionalism can be split into four distinct elements: being a digital advocate, using digital in a professional way, using digital as a professional tool for the people we care for, and using digital as a professional tool to support ourselves. By expanding on each of these elements we can start to form a picture of what digital professionalism looks like in nursing (Fig 4.1).

Being a digital advocate

In 2016, the Royal College of Nursing (RCN) at the RCN Congress 'agreed that the organisation (RCN) should lobby for every nurse to be

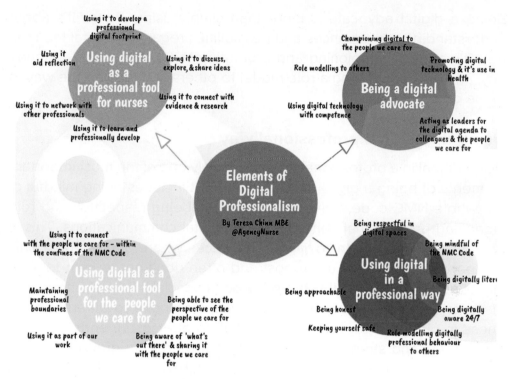

Figure 4.1   Elements of Digital Professionalism.

an e-nurse, able to use data, information, knowledge and technology to maximum effect for patients, carers and service users. These are no longer specialist issues but affect the whole nursing profession, who need to be supported to practise in new and modern ways' (RCN 2018). Every Registered Nurse has a responsibility to use digital technology and communication in their practice, which is why one of the elements of digital professionalism is being a digital advocate.

NMC

THE CODE SAYS

'You assess need and deliver or advise on treatment, or give help (including preventative or rehabilitative care) without too much delay and to the best of your abilities, on the basis of the best evidence available and best practice'

Being a digital advocate is more than simply using digital; it's about understanding the advances and possibilities regarding digital technology, it's about championing and promoting the use of digital technology, and it's about being a role model to others and leading the way in terms of digital.

Using digital in a professional way

Using digital in a professional way is arguably one of the most important elements of being a digital professional, as it includes being mindful of the whole NMC code, being approachable, being respectful, and role modelling professional behaviour in all digital communications. This is particularly important in social media spaces where often people only see part of a conversation or post and often don't get to hear tone or inflection. In addition to this there is also the social media phenomenon of context collapse 'Before social media, we spoke to different audiences in different ways. The way we talk to our close friends, parents, colleagues, and strangers is different — moving from group to group, we adjust our presentation to fit the context. However, online, with lists of followers in the thousands, our audience becomes challenging to address as a whole' (Bartz 2020) Speaking up and advocating for others is a necessary and important element of nursing. Complying with the Code and being an accountable professional does not mean we remain timid or hold back on our duty to challenge the status quo and create healthy, evidence-based debate within digital spaces. Digital communication, however, is challenging and it is something nursing students need to be mindful of in regard to digital professionalism and why being kind and respectful online is paramount.

Using digital as a professional tool to support the people we care for

Using digital as a professional tool to support the people we care for is fundamental to digital professionalism. The RCN (2018) states that digitally enabled health and social care services create improved outcomes for patients, better experiences for staff, and more efficient ways of working. There are always new and emerging technologies that can enhance the lives of the people we care for and as Registered Nurses and nursing students we need to be open to and aware of these technologies and their potential. In the RCN 'Every nurse is an e-nurse' (2018) consultation examples that specifically identified improvements in patient outcomes included:

- A digital photography app and accompanying database to improve the assessment and management of wounds following cardiothoracic surgery
- The introduction of telehealth to support patients with long-term conditions, enabling remote nursing triage
- Digital patient diaries in critical care, empowering families visiting patients to document their comments and concerns
- Texting services and websites for young people to discuss health issues
- An app to help inpatients manage their diabetes

Digital technology is a tool that plays a vital role in supporting the people we care for and as such we need an enhanced awareness of digital nursing. We also need to use digital technology professionally by applying the four core principles of the code (prioritise people, practise effectively, preserve safety, promote professionalism and trust), ensuring these technologies are safe and evidence-based and we act within our competencies. Digital competency and professionalism can be achieved by working closely with MDTs and employers and drawing on up-to-date evidence. The NHS England website, for example, provides service user links to apps selected by clinical policy teams that meet required technical and safety standards (nhs.uk, n.d. 2).

Using digital as a professional tool to support ourselves

Part of Registered Nurses and nursing students using digital as a professional tool to support themselves is the idea of creating a positive digital footprint. Students are often well versed in the concept of digital footprints but usually with negative connotations – how often have you heard someone advise you to stay anonymous online or not to share things publicly? Our lives are becoming increasingly integrated with our digital spaces, and everywhere we go on the world wide web we leave a digital footprint which is often seen as a bad thing, something we should be cautious of, something we need to be mindful of, and perhaps even strive to eradicate. Perhaps it's time to start looking at digital footprints in a different way? By not engaging in digital environments nursing students are potentially limiting their reputations and the reputations of their organisations. What would happen if you Googled an organisation and found nothing? It would be unusual, wouldn't it? So what happens when we Google an individual and find nothing? Does this also ring some alarm bells?

A lack of positive professional digital footprint could be a hindrance for a nursing student who eventually wants to become a working registrant and be open to opportunities and employers

CASE STUDY

Since 2014 the University of Plymouth have been preparing nursing students to work in the health and social care systems of the future by ensuring they have a broad base of clinical, professional, and personal skills that allow them to adapt to new situations. The PUNC Project (Plymouth University nursing Cohort) aims to enable students to be digitally professional. All first-year nursing students at the University of Plymouth are introduced to the use of Twitter and are asked to set up their own Twitter account; many opt to have PUNC somewhere in their Twitter name and include a statement in their 'BIO' that they are University of Plymouth nursing students (Jones 2016). Students and the university work in collaboration with@ WeNurses (a community of Registered Nurses on Twitter) to explore digital professionalism via a platform that embraces and uses social media in order to help students learn.

The project has led to an increased understanding of how digital and social media fits into nursing practice which can be seen from the

CASE STUDY—cont'd

pre- and post-course reflection question results. Students were asked the following questions to University of Plymouth nursing students both before starting the course and upon completion:

- How good is your knowledge of what digital professionalism is in nursing? (1 being no knowledge)
- How good is your knowledge of how digital professionalism can be used to aid development in nursing? (1 being no knowledge)
- How would you rate your skills in the use of Twitter? (1 being no skill)
- How would you rate your ability to use different types of social media? (1 being no ability)
- How much do you share learning, information, and resources that you have found online? (1 being no sharing)
- How good is your knowledge of the elements of digital professionalism in nursing? (1 being no knowledge)

The graph below shows how students responded before starting the course (the blue line) and upon completion (black line); it is clear to see the improvement made.

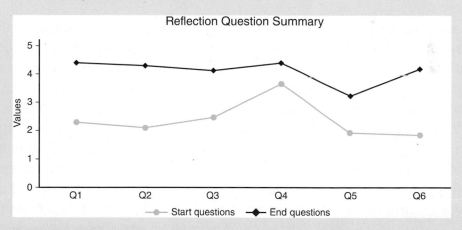

Nursing students were also asked to anonymously share feedback. One student who was part of the 2021 course stated, 'If I am being totally honest I rarely use social media and have little interest for it.

Continued

CASE STUDY—cont'd

However engaging with this platform it has shown me I am missing out on endless of opportunities. I feel twitter is a platform that healthcare professionals can feel comfortable engaging with and how important it to reach out to others and staying connected. I've enjoyed the potential elements of digital professionalism and being aware of how to create a positive digital footprint. Also I've learnt being able to use social media gives you the opportunity to promote health and well-being, communicating with other healthcare professionals, exchanging ideas and building on evidence informed decision making, providing patients with better care, and how we can use this in every day practise and always adhering to the NMC code in everything that we do'

Students gained so much from being aware of digital professionalism and how to use digital and social media to inform and support and as part of nursing practice.

To an extent, nursing students need to be mindful of the footprints they leave in digital spaces but we need to remember we are in control of our digital footprints; they are not something that simply 'happen'. Nursing students can craft and nurture positive professional digital footprints (Fig 4.2). By engaging professionally in social media spaces, writing blogs, appearing in videos, and commenting on articles, nursing students can use digital spaces to help them to build networks and professionally develop and advance their careers as Registered Nurses. It is good practice to work closely with your academic advisor and university communications team as they can guide you in this process as you learn how to communicate and portray yourself as a future Registered Nurses in a professional way.

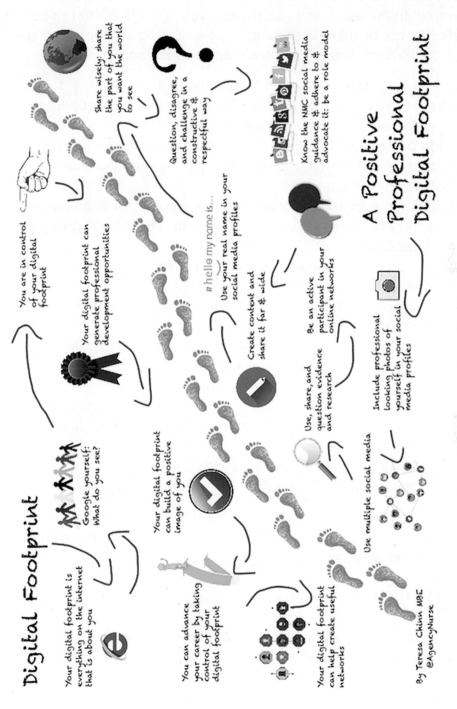

Figure 4.2 Digital Footprint.

The first step is for nursing students to see how the world sees them and 'Google' themselves and ask themselves, 'Do I like what I see?' If the answer is no, or there is nothing to see, nursing students can start to shape their digital footprints; some top tips include:

- Use your real name for social media accounts – yes, this is contrary to what we teach our children but this is about people seeing you and creating a positive digital footprint
- Include professional-looking photos as your avatars – again contrary to what we are often taught to do but remember that this is a professional space
- Using multiple forms of digital communication – for example, using Twitter and writing a blog or setting up a Facebook group and a YouTube Channel
- Use evidence and research in your digital spaces – don't leave evidence at the door just because it's digital
- Be an active participant in your online networks – jump in, join in, ask questions, talk to your peers
- Create content – write blogs, make videos, create infographics, etc.
- Share the part of you that you want the world to see – remember you are in control of your digital footprint
- Feel free to question, disagree, and challenge in a constructive and respectful way – it is possible to disagree and still remain professional
- Know the NMC Social Media Guidance (2019), adhere to it, and advocate professionalism online – be an active role model

Whilst nursing students need to be cautious, they also need to be courageous, taking positive steps and crafting digital footprints which can be both empowering and advantageous for individuals, organisations, and nursing.

SOCIAL MEDIA

There are many different groups, support, and resources within social media that nursing students can benefit from, but it's often difficult to know where to start. Social media is wide and diverse and prior to becoming a nursing student it may never have entered your thoughts that social media can be anything other than a place to connect with friends, follow celebrities, or learn how to fix your toaster! Here are some top social media accounts to follow and get involved with:

Twitter

@WeNurses and@WeStudentNurses – Communities of Registered Nurses who encourage learning and support through making connections with peers. Both accounts hold regular Twitter discussions that encourage people from all areas of nursing to come together to learn, develop, and grow.

@TeamCNO – The Chief Nursing Officer for England's team account advocating that all nursing, midwifery, and care staff have a key contribution to make to the delivery of the Long Term Plan.

The Chief Nursing Officers for each of the four countries across the UK also have Twitter accounts: @CNOWales @CNO_NI @CNOEngland @profalexmcmahon.

@OHID – Official feed of the Office for Health Improvement and Disparities. Working to improve the nation's health and reduce health disparities.

@theRCN – The Twitter account for the Royal College of Nursing, who are a trade union and professional body with close to half a million Registered Nurses, Midwives, HCA, AP, and student members.

@UNISONStudentNetwork – Twitter account for UNISON, who are a trade union for nursing students and AHP/wider NHS family, the largest in the UK.

@NMCnews – The Twitter account for the Nursing and Midwifery Council, who are the professional regulator of almost 748,000 nursing and midwifery professionals.

YouTube

NHS England and NHS Improvement – NHS England and NHS Improvement YouTube Channels that contain lots of resources to help support health and care professionals and the people we care for.

NHS Education for Scotland – The YouTube Channel for the education body within NHS Scotland.

The Kings Fund – YouTube Channel for The Kings Fund, who are an independent charitable organisation working to improve health and care in England.

khanacademymedicine – Easy-to-understand videos that explain every aspect of health and care.

Podcasts

Nursing Matters – A podcast from the RCN.

WePods – A podcast aimed at Registered Nurses and nursing students from the WeNurses and WeStudentNurses communities.

Anthony's Nursing Podcast (Anchor) – A podcast from a newly Registered Nurse.

'I developed my own nursing podcast in October 2020. My thinking behind the podcast was to bring the nursing community together in challenging times as we were in the middle of a global pandemic. At the time of writing this, I have 16 episodes. I have had a variety of guests from a teacher, nursing students, re-deployed staff, Registered Nurses from the charity sector, celebrity fitness trainers, and my most recent one, which I'm incredibly proud of, is our Chief Nursing Officer for England, Ruth May.

In my podcast, I have covered a wide range of topics relevant to the nursing community. Language and communication, ICU experience during the pandemic, Nursing Students COVID experience, the importance of reflective practice, role of the clinical nurse tutor, a leadership series, benefits of exercise for your physical and mental health and dyslexia within nursing.

I have found my podcast as a good but simple way to share best practice within nursing. As I have a good following and reputation on twitter and I'm also in a very privileged position of being part of team @WeNurses I have found that I can use my position to be a *role model for young Registered Nurses coming through and try to inspire the whole nursing community. It's very important to always stay digitally professional.*

In my leadership series, I have found a massive benefit for myself getting to know and talking to students and Registered Nurses all over the world. I have learnt so much from each individual I have spoken to on my podcast and I think it's amazing I can share this learning with the whole nursing community worldwide through social media.

I think it is fantastic we can celebrate and share nursing practice through podcasts and social media in such a simple way, something I can only encourage people to get involved in. If you are a nursing students or a very experienced Registered Nurse, get involved on social media you would be surprised how much you can learn from others!'

–Anthony Swan, Registered Nurse

Facebook

Royal College of Nursing Libraries – The official Facebook page of the RCN Library.

NursingNotes – The Facebook page of the open-access nursing news website Nursing Notes.

NIHR – The Facebook page for the National Institute for Health Research.

Instagram

Cochrane_uk – The Instagram account of the UK Cochrane Centre, who share trusted health and care-based evidence and research.

Protectnurse – A campaign to make nurse and protected title in UK law.

Foundation_of_nursing_studies – A non-profit organisation who work with nurse-led health and social care teams to develop and share ways of improving practice and to create person-centred, safe, and effective cultures.

WHO – The Instagram account for the World Health Organization.

Social media and fitness to practice

Let's explore the area of fitness to practise from a regulator's perspective to help dispel some myths or misguided fear that may still prevail amongst peers.

As part of the research for this chapter, a meeting was held with the NMC to request data on social media referrals and better understand how investigations into registrants' fitness to practice are triaged. An NMC Report (2022) was subsequently produced with some very helpful and interesting statistics.

From 2017 to 2021, 82% of social media referrals to the NMC were made by members of the public (MoP) or anonymous referrers. There was also a notable spike during the 2020/21 pandemic lockdowns (Fig 4.3).

The most common outcome was not to investigate, as the referral did not meet the NMC's threshold. Why do you think this might be? One of the key findings of the report is that concerns relating to social media seemed to be reflective of external or environmental factors rather than indicators of risk to patient or public safety (NMC 2022) (Fig 4.4).

The NMC's role is to decide whether a Registered Nurse is meeting the NMC Code and professional standards. What this data highlights is that ongoing work needs to be done to educate the general public on what the role of the NMC as regulator for the profession is. Cases that do not meet the NMC threshold for investigation are filtered out at the triage stage

When cases are investigated, the NMC always considers context. For example:

- Accidental confidentiality breach (e.g. a selfie background) versus intentional breach (disclosure of a diagnosis online).
- The RN's response to an allegation, for example, demonstrates understanding and is reflective versus being defensive, argumentative, and unreflective.

Referral Trend Spikes on social media include:

- Racial Discrimination
- Social Distancing breaches
- Vaccination Views/Covid-19 Misinformation

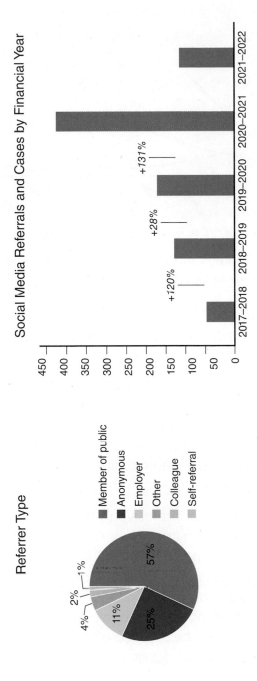

Referrer Type

Member of public
Anonymous
Employer
Other
Colleague
Self-referral

57%
25%
11%
4%
2%
1%

Members of the public (MoP) are the most common referrer type, accounting for 57% of these types of referrals. However, when this is combined with the second most common referrer type, it is found that MoP and anonymous referrers account collectively for 82% of these types of referrals.

Social Media Referrals and Cases by Financial Year

2017–2018   2018–2019   2019–2020   2020–2021   2021–2022

+120%   +28%   +131%

450
400
350
300
250
200
150
100
50
0

The number of referrals and cases involving social media allegations has been continuing to rise for each financial year, including before the pandemic. Initial referral rates from the beginning of the financial year of 2021–2022 indicate that the spike will not be repeated, but that the numbers are still higher than pre-pandemic levels.

Figure 4.3 Social Media Referrals and Cases by Month From 01 April 2017 to 18 November 2021. (Source: NMC, 2022).

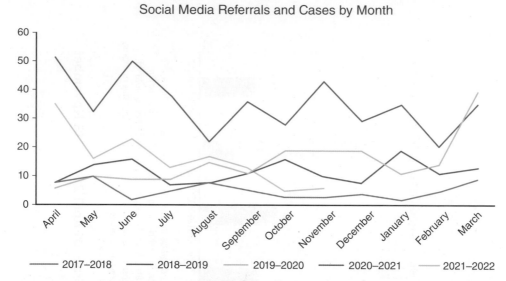

Figure 4.4   **Quantitative Findings of Analysis of Social Media Referrals and Cases** From 01 April 2017 to 18 November 2021.

The NMC analysis notes that 'other categories have fluctuated between 2017 and 2021, but Discrimination or Intolerance has seen a consistent year-on-year increase of over 100%' (NMC 2021).

Expression of a view that is discriminatory or shows intolerance towards others clearly impacts your ability to promote trust or develop therapeutic and professional working relationships within your nursing role. Nursing Education includes such topics and it is important that students translate this learning into practice within digital spaces as future registrants and digital professionals.

The NMC's role is not to act as our profession's moral police. Whilst this perception may have been rooted in an era when Registered Nurses were confined to nurse quarters, our profession and autonomy has evolved since. The NMC is only interested in cases that indicate risk to patient or public safety or which could damage public confidence in the professions. Rest assured, however, that being professional, kind, and respectful in your activities on digital platforms helps ensure you adhere to the NMC code and act as advocates for the profession you aspire to step into.

There is a really helpful NMC series of videos entitled Caring with Confidence (2020), which have a video specifically aimed at social media and can be found on the NMC's web site.

MYTH BUSTING

Despite the growing and widespread use of digital platforms, far too many myths and misguided information exist about their use in nursing. If you were held to account for breaching patient confidentiality during a conversation with a fellow student on a bus, would you stop using the bus? We hope not! Instead you would learn from the experience, modify your behaviour, and continue to use the bus. It is important not to blame digital platforms but instead learn how to use them professionally. Negative messaging that instils fear rather than knowledge on how to become digitally professional persists and can be unhelpful.

MYTH – Digital spaces are full of trolls

MYTH PARTIALLY BUSTED – We are sorry to say that trolls – people that 'hide behind their computers or phones, and go out of their way to cause misery online' (BBC 2019) – exist. There are people in digital spaces that troll others; however, this is something that we need to put into context – trolls are the minority, not the majority. Most people use digital spaces in a kind, productive, and compassionate way. Devon and Cornwall Police (2022) suggest taking the following action if you do encounter a troll online:

- Do not respond to the troll
- Block the troll
- Change your privacy setting
- Tell someone such as a family member or a friend
- Always report the abuse to the social network or site owner
- Keep a record of any aggressive or intimidating messages, posts, pictures, or videos you receive or see
- If the abuse is really serious – report it to the police

MYTH – Digital spaces are bad for your mental health

MYTH PARTIALLY BUSTED – There is mixed opinion and evidence around digital spaces and mental health, Scott et al. (2017) state that society's use of technology has negative consequences including lowered social skills, self-motivation, emotional intelligence, empathy and increased conflict with others, ADHD, and depression in younger populations. Whereas Haidt and Allen (2020) suggest that 'perhaps digital devices could provide a way of gathering data about mental health in a systematic way, and make interventions more timely' With the evidence being mixed it's vital in nursing we are mindful of the potential effects of digital technology on our mental health by taking a purposeful and productive approach to digital spaces. In relation to social media it's worth periodically asking yourself these questions (Bashforth 2021):

- How do I feel when I am using social media?
- Does it make me angry, happy, sad, or anxious?
- Am I grinding my teeth and struggling to sleep?
- Does what I see on social media influence my mood?
- Is my social media usage interfering with my day-to-day life?

MYTH – Nursing students should not publicise their identity on social media or they should lock down their social media accounts for fear of possible litigation or fitness to practice hearings

MYTH BUSTED – Think about this. Technology is smart and being anonymous is not a protection from litigation. It's also crucial to remember that all social media can be duplicated, copied, and redistributed; therefore, locking down accounts is not a safeguard. The best course of action is to always be professional; that way you won't find yourself in trouble.

The NMC social media guidance (2019) states, 'it is important to realise that even the strictest privacy settings have limitations. This is because, once something is online, it can be copied and redistributed'.

MYTH – Social media platforms are unprofessional and nursing students should stay away from them

MYTH BUSTED – There are many nursing students using social media in a very professional way. It's important to remember that social media platforms are not unprofessional; it's how we use them in nursing that constitutes being professional or unprofessional.

CONCLUSION

Ultimately there are advantages and disadvantages to using digital spaces and digital tools in nursing. However, if nursing students remain digitally professional then the pros far outweigh the cons. Being digitally professional is ultimately professionalism applied in digital spaces and in nursing we need to think of digital spaces as an extension of our workplaces applying the same thinking and behaviours. The benefits that come from being online and digitally savvy in nursing are huge, so the way we conduct ourselves in these spaces and the way that we use digital with and for the people we care for is a significant issue for nursing students to get to grips with.

Now, that you have finished this chapter. Make some notes on what you have learned.

_____

_____

_____

_____

_____

_____

_____

_____

_____

_____

_____

_____

_____

_____

_____

_____

_____

_____

REFERENCES

Bartz, J. (2020) *Social media and the effects of context collapse* [online] Available at: https://jasonmbartz.medium.com/understanding-context-collapse-and-the-restoration-of-our-walled-gardens-1325bf527cf [Accessed 26/8/22].

Bashforth, E. (2021) *How to look after your mental health on social media* [online] Available at: https://patient.info/news-and-features/how-to-look-after-your-mental-health-on-social-media [Accessed 26/8/22].

BBC (2019) *Why do people troll and what you can do about it* [online] Available at: https://www.bbc.co.uk/bitesize/articles/zfmkrj6 [Accessed 26/8/22].

Devon & Cornwall Police (2022) *What is trolling (cyber bullying)* [online] Available at: https://www.devon-cornwall.police.uk/advice/your-digital-safety/what-is-trolling/ [Accessed 26/8/22].

Gov.UK (2014) *Personalised health and care 2020* [online] Available at: https://www.gov.uk/government/publications/personalised-health-and-care-2020 [Accessed 30/8/2022].

Haidt, J. & Allen, N. (2020) *Scrutinizing the effects of digital technology on mental health* [online] Available at: https://www.nature.com/articles/d41586-020-00296-x [Accessed 26/8/22].

McKinsey & Company (2015). *What 'digital' really means* [online] Available at: https://www.mckinsey.com/industries/technology-media-and-telecommunications/our-insights/what-digital-really-means [Accessed 26/8/22].

NHS England (2021) *Making research matter: Chief Nursing Officer for England's strategic plan for research* [online] Available at: https://www.england.nhs.uk/publication/making-research-matter-chief-nursing-officer-for-englands-strategic-plan-for-research/ [Accessed 30/8/2022].

NHS England (2022) *Wellbeing apps* [online] Available at: https://www.england.nhs.uk/supporting-our-nhs-people/support-now/wellbeing-apps/ [Accessed 30/8/2022].

NHSx (2022) *Driving forward the digital transformation of health and social care* Available at: https://www.nhsx.nhs.uk/ [Accessed 30/8/2022].

NMCVideos (2020) Let's talk about social media | Caring with Confidence: The Code in Action | NMC Available at: https://youtu.be/lJodYFg_JFg (Accessed 27/03/2023)

Nursing & Midwifery Council (2017) *Enabling professionalism in nursing and midwifery practice.*

Nursing & Midwifery Council (2018) *The Code: Professional standards of practice and behaviour for nurses, midwives and nursing associates.*

Nursing & Midwifery Council (2019) *Social media guidance* [online] Available at: https://www.nmc.org.uk/standards/guidance/social-media-guidance/ [Accessed 30/8/2022].

Nursing & Midwifery Council (2022) *Social media analysis: 01 April 2017–18 November 2021* [Accessed 30/9/2022].

Royal College of Nursing (2018) *Every nurse an E-nurse: Insights from a consultation on the digital future of nursing* [online] Available at: https://www.rcn.org.uk/professional-development/publications/pdf-007013 [Accessed 26/8/22].

Scott, D.A., Valley, B. & Simecka, B.A. (2017) Mental Health Concerns in the Digital Age. *Int J Ment Health Addict* 15, 604–613.

WHO (2021) *Global strategy on digital health 2020–2025* [online] Available at: https://apps.who.int/iris/bitstream/handle/10665/344249/9789240020924-eng.pdf [Accessed 30/8/2022].

TWITTER REFERENCES

Ball, P. (2022) [Twitter] 21/2/22 Available at: https://twitter.com/PhilBallRN/status/1495853496813375491?s=20&t=kPhP8HIgARHqS931nD-hww [Accessed 26/8/22].

Chinn, T. (2019) The elements of digital professioanlism. Twitter [Online Image] Available from: https://twitter.com/WeNurses/status/1087730685329264643?s=20 [Accessed 27/03/2023]

Jakab-Hall, C. (2022) [Twitter] 22/2/22 Available at: https://twitter.com/CharlotteNI ISRN/status/1495967685947101186?s=20&t=kPhP8HIgARHqS931nD-hww [Accessed 26/8/22].

Jones, R. (2016) *University of Plymouth Nursing Cohorts (@PUNC on Twitter)* [online] Available at: https://www.plymouth.ac.uk/schools/school-of-nursing-and-midwifery/punc [Accessed 26/8/22].

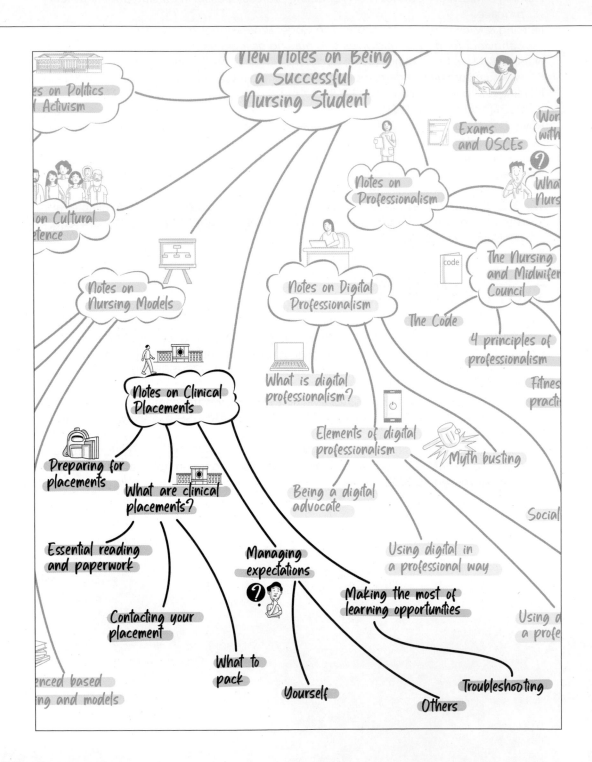

NOTES ON CLINICAL PLACEMENTS

Natalie Elliott (She/Her) ■ Simon James (He/Him)

INTRODUCTION

In the UK, a minimum of 2,300 of clinical placement hours are required to be completed for a nursing student to be deemed competent for entry to the NMC register. This has been set by EU law.

> 'The training of nurses responsible for general care shall comprise a total of at least three years of study, which may in addition be expressed with the equivalent ECTS credits, and shall consist of at least 4,600 hours of theoretical and clinical training, the duration of the theoretical training representing at least one third and the duration of the clinical training at least one half of the minimum duration of the training. Member States may grant partial exemptions to professionals who have received part of their training on courses which are of at least an equivalent level'.

– Article 31 of 2005/36/EC EU Law

The below Twitter poll shows that placement tends to be 67% the part of the course that nursing students look forward to the most. It is a time when you are able to link the theory learned to the reality of delivering care and hopefully this is where things begin to make sense.

Whilst clinical placements are the most anticipated aspect of the course, they can be one of the most anxiety-producing aspects of a student's journey (Watt et al., 2016); therefore, it is hoped that the contents of this chapter will help you feel more prepared.

The Nursing and Midwifery Council (NMC), has an expectation that students will encounter a variety of placements involving a range of shift patterns which covers different clinical settings. This means that nursing students can experience many different clinical areas to consolidate their learning through practice. It's also important that nursing students have experience in caring for people across the lifespan and covering all fields of practice. As an example, an adult field nursing student will be expected to understand caring for children, mental health patients, people with learning disabilities, and pregnant women.

Clinical placements providers assume equal responsibilty with the Approved Educational Institue to ensure the nursing student gains a wide variety of clinical experience to aid their development. The settings can range from the local health board/trust hospitals and community locations) to private clinics, social care settings, prisons, GP surgeries, schools, and many more places. This enables the student to experience a variety of areas where nursing care is provided to all different types of patients.

> 'They must be able to care for people in their own home, in
> the community or hospital or in any health care settings
> where their needs are supported and managed'. NMC Future
> Nurse Proficiencies

Placements are a great opportunity to implement what you have learned at university into the clinical environment. It's not just clinical skills that you will get to practice but you will also be able to apply the theoretical side of things. Placements are essential to building the skills and knowledge needed to gain entry into the NMC register.

TWEET

@nikkilouh

'To learn in a practical way in order to put theory into practice. To experience different experiences to decide which fits for you, to learn skills you can't get in text books, to work with wider teams and professionals and to develop yourself and the nurse you want to be'

Not only do nursing students learn from experiences in clinical placements, but students can use these experiences to deepen their learning and enhance their emotional intelligence through reflection, which will be discussed later in the chapter. Registered Nurses face emotional strain within their job, especially when caring for people who are experiencing challenging situations; therefore, improving emotional intelligence aids Registered Nurses in delivering high-quality and balanced care (Mansel and Einion, 2019). Additionally, clinical experience will allow you to bring situations back from practice to inform class discussions.

CASE STUDY

Ahmed, a year 3 nursing student, was on placement in an acute gastroenterology ward. One of the patients, an 85-year-old lady who is living with dementia and receiving palliative care due to cervical cancer, was receiving end-of-life care and there was a conflict between the medical staff and the patient's family as to the best course of treatment. She was admitted from a hospice and had minimal nutritional intake for 3 weeks. Hospice staff tried on several occasions to insert a nasal-gastric tube; however, this was not tolerated by her. Therefore, she presented to a gastroenterology ward for the insertion of a percutaneous endoscopic gastrostomy (PEG) as she became cachexic, which is a commonly associated complication of dementia. Due to the dementia diagnosis, she had an Adults With Incapacity (AWI) order in place which safeguards the welfare and managing of finances of adults who lack capacity. The nursing staff

Continued

CASE STUDY—cont'd

are against the procedure as they feel that it is unethical to prolong life without meaningful quality. However, the family are keen to proceed believing that it would be the wishes of the patient; staff are unsure if this is a decision based on and influenced by their own wishes or if it is a true depiction of her wishes.

At the time the scenario took place, Ahmed had little understanding of the rationale with which decisions were made; however, he did know that this was an ethical dilemma. When he returned to university, he used this experience to talk with his peers and lecturers to reflect and gain a deeper level of thinking.

Students often struggle with the uncertainty of clinical placements. Whilst on a theory block, classes are at set times, and you have a structure for the days and weeks. You are able to plan around this by making childcare, paid employment, or just having a social life (which is a rarity as a nursing student!) much easier.

When on placement you may not know which area you are going to be allocated until the last minute, or you might not get your shifts until the day you start, which makes life difficult to plan. There is the added challenge that healthcare is unpredictable in nature, in that patients can deteriorate quickly; it will be a steep learning curve to learn new conditions or communication methods that perhaps haven't been covered in class. You may have no experience of healthcare and are a little unsure how to manage your expectations and those of others. But please have faith; you can get through this.

Flexibility is highly important. Being open to new opportunities and being prepared to reconsider planned learning activities in the event of unplanned events is a key skill to develop as a Registered Nurse, as not every day is the same. This will enable you to learn to think on your feet and prioritise your workload.

FIRST PLACEMENT

What are your worries and your hopes for your upcoming placement?

_____

_____

_____

_____

_____

_____

_____

Preparing for placements

The email has finally arrived in the inbox and the excitement and anxiety begins to build ... the first placement destination is revealed! Being prepared for a clinical placement is essential and will help you set off on the correct trajectory. Being prepared will also help with some of the nerves. Below are some handy tips to get you placement ready.

> 'By failing to prepare, you are preparing to fail'.
>
> **– Benjamin Franklin**

Essential reading before starting your first clinical placement

Before starting placement, it is good practice to refresh yourself with some of the recommended reading. It will show your placement area that you are professional, conscientious, and enthusiastic – which will get you off to a good start.

- NMC Code
- NMC Standards of Proficiency for Registered Nurses
- Importance of informed consent

- Confidentiality and data protection – for your university and for your NHS Trust
- Uniform policy – for your university and for your NHS Trust
- Social media policy
- Research the common conditions found in the area you will be learning

Contacting the placement

First impressions count, so it's important to think about how to contact the placement. Students often struggle and become anxious with this, especially if they have any special requests about needing particular days off. Be as flexible and respectful as possible; however, if there are unavoidable commitments then be forthcoming and allow them time to plan ahead. Your placement will be aware of where there are opportunities to maximise your learning, so it's important to make sure you try every opportunity to progress from your placement.

Speaking on the phone to someone new can be a nerve-wracking experience. The excitement levels will almost definitely mean panic sets in, and priorities will be forgotten. When asking for a rota, a common response from staff could be, 'just turn up on the first day and we'll sort it'. This can be anxiety-provoking for some students, particularly if you have commitments that you need to work around. However, under the new Standards of Proficiency (NMC, 2018a, b, or c) students are able to work with any member of staff, not only their practice supervisor or assessor, so flexibility around rotas should be granted; however, many placements will expect you to work alongside a member of staff as students should not be left unsupervised.

Asking about the uniform policy is a good idea. Whilst most of the acute settings will require you to wear a uniform, some areas prefer you to wear smart clothes or casual business attire (e.g. Health Visiting), so asking for clarity on this is worthwhile.

Preparing a list of things that you want to talk about before making the phone call is helpful. If you find it difficult to make contact via the telephone due to the placement being busy, it's also worth thinking about sending an email. It's good to do as early as you can to give the staff time to respond.

 TIP

Here is a sample script you may wish to use for contacting placement that you can tailor to your needs and give you an idea of what you might want to include.

Hello, my name is XXXX and I am a XX year nursing student from XXXX. Could I please speak with XXXX.

I am very excited to start placement here on XXX and I'm wondering if now is convenient for me to ask some questions?

I was wondering if you are able to give me my rota, along with the start and finish times. Will I be expected to work night shift or weekends? I have children, so it would be helpful to know so that I can arrange childcare.

I have some commitments during my placement, and I was wondering if it would be possible not to be rostered for XXXX.

Will I be expected to wear my uniform?

Do I have allocated practice assessor and supervisor?

Can you tell me about the catering facilities? Will I have access to a microwave, hot water, canteen?

Is there anything you would like me to do to prepare for starting and do you have an induction booklet?

Thank you very much for your time; I look forward to meeting you and the team on XXXX.

Uniform

If you have to wear a uniform on placement, make sure you pack this. Whilst there is no evidence of an infection risk from travelling in uniform, many people perceive it to be unhygienic and therefore it is deemed good practice to change into and out of uniform at work (NHS Employers, 2020). It is worth considering buying (or making – if you are the creative type) a uniform bag so it can go straight into the washing machine when you get home – especially important for infection control purposes. A uniform bag is a cloth bag that you can pop your uniform into once you have finished your shift. When you get home, you can throw the bag and its contents straight into the washing machine so that any germs from your uniform don't contaminate the other items in your household.

Name badge

Although you should always be wearing your name badge, it's also important to introduce yourself to each patient you meet for the first time (or those who may need a little reminding). Wearing a name badge is important to identify who you are and to inform people of your name.

The '#hellomynameis' campaign was developed in 2013 by Dr Kate Granger (Granger, 2013). Dr Granger was terminally ill at the time and noticed that those looking after her didn't introduce themselves to her before delivering care. Not only is it common courtesy to introduce yourself to someone new, but introductions help form human connections between one who is vulnerable and in need of help and another who wishes to help. This is how the power barrier is broken down and trusting therapeutic relationships can start to build.

Footwear

A very common question amongst nursing students is which trainers or shoes they should buy for clinical placement. There is no set answer to this and it's down to the individual. Some key considerations should be given to:

- Material type. Leather footwear (in the colour recommended in your local uniform policy) are recommended. You may be assisting patients with showers, or who are incontinent, so leather will keep your feet dry!

- Try to have a specific pair of placement trainers or shoes due to infection control.
- Consider your budget – don't go bargain basement but then don't blow all your student finance on a pair of shoes!
- Comfort – you may be on your feet for a very long time, so it's important to focus on whether they are comfortable and not just aesthetically pleasing.
- Durability – these trainers or shoes will need to last a long time, so it's important to consider if they will be able to withstand the test of time.
- Your feet – everyone has differently shaped feet, and one size does not fit all. Consider if you have any special requirements.

Nursing kit

A fob watch and pen torch. The fob watch will allow you to count heart rates and respiratory rates. A pen torch is handy not only for doing neurological observations but also if you are doing night shift and need a torch for the dark! It may be worth asking if you can take your stethoscope and sphygmomanometer to practice your manual blood pressure skills.

It is a good idea to have a few black pens and possibly a red pen to note important things you want to learn more about or to write things you need to do. A notebook is also useful to add anything you have learned and to make note of questions you might have, conditions you want to research, and abbreviations you come across – healthcare professionals use them a lot!

If you are asked to wear a face mask in practice, it can get hot underneath, so a good lip balm is important to prevent lips from becoming chapped. You will also be performing hand hygiene frequently throughout the day, so skin care is vital, and a good hand cream will be useful to have in your pocket.

What will you pack in your bag ready for placement?

_____

_____

_____

_____

_____

_____

Placement paperwork

It goes without saying, but please remember to pack your paperwork and that you have completed what is relevant to this placement. It's also recommended to make yourself familiar with the learning outcomes you need to achieve.

Food and drink

You may be doing a 12-hour-shift and it can be expensive to buy food for every meal, especially on a student budget, so consider taking your food in with you. Batch cooking on your day off is an excellent way to ensure you are saving money and eating healthily – you will also be glad to have done it in advance. The last thing you will feel like doing after a long shift is cook. Some suggestions have been given below – and remember to invest in good plastic food containers to prevent spillages.

TWEET

@mozzaedwards:

'Baked potatoes done in a microwave look different to oven baked, but split filled with cheese, scrambled egg, houmous or beans are cheap and fill'

TWEET

@SarahLouiseJ:

'This is literally fresh pasta (can use dry I do when I'm short on money), turkey breast (I use chicken if it's cheaper and free what's left), crème fresh, parmesan and Italian spices. Its such a cheap meal and if you have stuff left can make something else'

TWEET

@SarahSt51234485:

'I lived on pasta, chopped up ham and pesto on placements! Can be eaten hot or cold'

TWEET

@SarahLouiseJ:

'Soup as well. My god what a life saver. If you ever have any spare money get a soup maker. I throw everything in the fridge in it so nothing goes to watse'

TWEET

@SimonJa39523855:

'grains/noodles and cold meat with some sauce over the top'

TWEET

@Stew77Laura:

'Big batch of any veg roasted then added to pasta, cous cous, wraps, top with grated cheese, cottage cheese, sweet chilli sauce, pesto, delicious hot or cold and make enough for 3 x 12 hour shifts'

TWEET

@kayleighmmanley:

'Anything that can be batch cooked! Pasta bakes, chilli, curries, soups (butternut squash and sage is a personal fav), paella's, jambalaya. And apart from pasta bakes, these can be frozen so I have a selection of meals to choose from'

TWEET

@BrianWebster18:

'I like to make an omelette (so a few eggs and then any choice of extras such as onions, tomatoes, anything really) and then pop the whole omelette onto a wrap. Its an amazing, cheap, quick breakfast (or any time meal) and feels like a fakeaway McDonalds Breakfast wrap'

TWEET

@sarah16107480:

'Batch cook at weekend. Satay noodles- pack of dried noodles, cooked. Stir fry onion carrot, cabbage, mushrooms, +/- tofu. Make sauce with peanut butter and chilli sauce, with a little water to thin it out. Divide into 5 portions and keep in fridge. Or couscous with roast veg and chicken or halloumi- can do a jar of roast veg or cook alongside something else. Cook chicken or other protein and divide up and mix with grated carrot/ cabbage/ apples and vinaigrette as a salad'

Nursing is a physically demanding profession, often involving shift work, walking for many miles, and short breaks, meaning it's important to stay hydrated. Dehydration affects your concentration and brain power, and it also leads to fatigue which can be deemed a potential risk to patients if we aren't working to our fullest capacity (El-Sharkawy et al., 2016).

Therefore, it's important to keep hydrated and investing in a water bottle to refill throughout the day is worthwhile.

Anything else

Anything that's specific to you, for example, medications, glasses, deodorant, hair ties, etc.

Checklist

What to pack for placement

- [ ] Uniform & name badge
- [ ] Leather trainers
- [ ] Pens and small notebook
- [ ] Hand cream and lip balm
- [ ] Placement paperwork
- [ ] Fab watch and pen torch
- [ ] Meals and snacks
- [ ] Fluids
- [ ]
- [ ]

Pre-reading

Enquiring if there's any preparatory reading or an induction booklet shows you are enthusiastic and conscientious. If you are given some preparatory work, remember to have it available for your first day, along with any questions you may have. Here are some places you could look for information, along with the reading already mentioned:

- The National Institute of Clinical Excellence (or NICE) or Scottish Intercollegiate Guidelines Network websites
- Charity websites that are associated with your speciality (e.g. Diabetes UK, British Heart Foundation, Mind etc).
- Cochrane Library
- University library to see what recent journal articles are available.

You will find that each clinical area you visit will have its own common medications, but here are some of the most generically used (why not make a start by finding out what they do and their side effects):

- Amoxicillin
- Aspirin
- Bisoprolol
- Buscopan (hyoscine butylbromide)
- Clopidogrel
- Codeine
- Cyclizine
- Diazepam
- Edoxaban
- Furosemide
- Hydrocortisone
- Lactulose
- Metformin
- Nystatin
- Omeprazole/lansoprazole
- Paracetamol
- Ramipril
- Senna
- Zopiclone

TIP

It can be difficult to pronounce some of the drug names – so Google Translate is your friend! Type the drug name into Google Translate and it should be able to give you the right pronunciation.

Paperwork

It's also important to complete the placement paperwork prior to stepping foot into the clinical arena. The university may ask you to produce an action plan of what you wish to achieve and how you plan to do this. During the course induction this should be explained and if there are any queries then the student's academic assessor is always a good port of call. You should follow your university's guidance on this. This section generally includes the interviews and competencies, and the practice assessor will detail, during your first interview, which they think is attainable.

Travel

Have you thought about how you plan on getting to your placement? Once you know where it is going to be, it is time to start thinking about how you are going to get there. It is important to take into account the local transport routes, the car parking situation, and how doing a range of shifts (or working on public holidays) will impact you. You are also going to want to think about the time of day that you will be travelling.

 'I had one placement where I was Monday to Friday, 9am until 5pm. Normally the journey would have only taken 30 minutes by car, but because I was travelling during the peak times, it took me well over an hour'.

– Natalie Elliott, registered nurse

Therefore, if possible, it's worth trialling the journey at the same time you will be travelling to placement. If you drive, it's also beneficial to scope out parking places. Please ensure you allocate time to get from the hospital grounds to the changing area and to the placement location. Some hospitals are huge, and it could add an extra 30 minutes to your travel time.

'I had a placement where the parking was free, but it was a 10-minute walk to the hospital from the car park so I had to factor this additional time into my travel time'.

– Simon James, registered nurse

And...relax

Undoubtedly you are going to be nervous, but it's important to try and rest the day before. Do the things you love, take a bath, go for a walk, pamper yourself, and try to get an early night. You may struggle to sleep but try your best to be well rested.

TWEET

@scPALMERNASH:

'I do like to have zero plans for the day before. I try and have no uni work to do or other to do list items. Just so I have a clear, well rested head. Probably a day of easy viewing boxset(s) and early night. If I am anxious, I might for go for a long(ish) drive as I find it relaxing'

TWEET

@KOHCltd:

'Nice walk somewhere, nice long bath and Netflix, listen to a podcast or music, spend time with family'

MANAGING YOUR NERVES

Nerves are completely natural when facing a new environment.

TWEET

@hpeveringham:

'I was absolutely terrified. I'd been placed on an ICU (covid=less student capacity) just as cases were picking up again last January. Luckily, they could all see I was bricking it so made me feel part of the team and supported the whole way! Mentors make the difference!'

It's fair to say that you have a big part to play in making the most of your placement. You could be a passive bystander who does the mini-mum, or you can take an active role in your learning and seek out opportunities.

'During clinical placements I find it important to remember that my success is dependent on myself. I am responsible for my learning, to know what I need to achieve and to seek out opportunities to do so. The nurses I work with have their qualification and a job to do each shift and I am there to learn. I push myself to be proactive, to ask others if I can observe or take part in skills that I need to practice. It's easy to sit and wait to be told what to do, but the feedback I've received from being active in my learning has been nothing but positive and constructive'.

— Terrie-Ann Wright, nursing student

Before you step through the door, stop, compose yourself, take a deep breath, and hold your head up high. Even though your nerves will be jangling, and you may be feeling imposter syndrome, as we've already mentioned first impressions count. Try to keep smiling through the nerves (and the face covering!), do your best to appear calm (some deep breaths will trick your brain into thinking everything is okay), and introduce yourself (#hellomynameis). Be clear about who you are, which university you are from, and which year you are in. If it's your first placement, make sure to tell them that. It's also okay to let them know you are nervous – they will have been students at one point too, so they will remember what it feels like.

The RCN have produced a series of videos called 'Time and space' to help Registered Nurses and nursing students prepare for each aspect of your day (RCN, 2021) which can be found online and are well worth exploring.

'I remember being so fresh and excited, smiling at all the staff (before covid) trying to make a good 1st impression.. it was actually rare that anyone smiled back, it made me feel so unwelcome taking a huge toll on my MH and confidence. As a third year I've learnt it's not a crime to smile, in fact it's SO important. I smile at everyone even if they don't smile back. I would never want to make anyone (esp 1st year STNs) feel the way I did in my first placement. It was never a reflection of me, and took me a while to realise that'

–Rachel Fairs, nursing student

Whatever you are feeling, remember that it's natural to have a variety of feelings, almost certainly before and during placement, ranging from positive to negative and somewhere in the middle. The important thing is to not let them define and hinder you. Acknowledge what you are feeling but don't allow it to consume you. Countless nursing students have endured this emotional rollercoaster; however, support is readily available from university, friends, and family- just reach out!

'My first placement was (unusually!) on A&E. It was a wonderful experience but it really made me question if this was the career for me. I was so nervous. Luckily I had some amazing support and came away feeling so proud of myself for making it through what was a challenge for me'

—Gemma Parry, nursing student

MANAGING EXPECTATIONS

While on placement, you will have supernumerary status. This means that you are there not just to observe but to learn how to deliver safe and effective care (NMC, 2018b). However, you should never be counted within the staffing numbers or be left unsupervised to do anything that is not within your competency level or that you have not been taught to do. If you find yourself in any of these positions, please politely speak up and let the staff know that you feel uncomfortable.

 TIP

It is also recommended to research the best practice on how a skill should be carried out. Here is an example of how you can do this:

This is something I have only observed/never done/before, and I don't really feel comfortable doing this on my own. I am really interested in learning how to do this correctly.

Would it be okay if I research the best practice on how to do this? Then it would be really helpful if you could talk me through how to do this/ observe me closely to help me increase my confidence.

It is key to be aware of your limitations and know when to ask for help — patient safety should be at the core. It would also be worthwhile emailing your link lecturer to keep them abreast of the situation if you are not being afforded a supernumerary status.

Being aware of the expectations first-year nursing students place upon themselves is something to be mindful of. As a first-year nursing student it's important to have realistic expectations in line with the level of training and sphere of competency.

TWEET
@PUNC20_Michelle:

'Speaking to my personal tutor at university, she advised me to go in and learn from every single staff member, regardless of their banding as they would all teach me at least one thing. The support from the faculty has been amazing at letting me know what has been expected in every placement so far and has helped to ease the immense pressure that I put on myself and allowed me to set realistic goals and to push myself a little bit more each time'

Managing your own expectations

The first year of a nursing degree can be a huge learning curve. It's essential to remember that for most students it means adjusting to new environments and for some new routines with shift start times that some have never experienced before. It's vital not to be too hard on yourself, this is a new situation, and you are not expected to know absolutely everything. Most veteran Registered Nurses will tell you that they don't know everything. The key is to know whom to ask or where to find the information if you are unsure of anything. On the one hand there is a craving to learn and excel, and on the other it's learning to adapt and survive. Be kind to yourself and try to go with the flow. It is very common to become emotional from the things witnessed in a clinical placement. Don't bottle it up – reach out, talk, and reflect.

Managing the expectation of practice assessors and practice supervisors

Whilst out on placement the nursing student will be assigned a practice assessor who is tasked with supporting them in their learning journey by means of accomplishing competencies and discussing progress through a series of interviews. Practice assessors (PA) evaluate and validate the student's achievement of practice learning for a placement or a series of placements (NMC, 2018). The practice supervisor's (PS's) role is to support and oversee students in the practice learning environment and feed back to the assessor (NMC, 2018). More recently, more flexibility has been achieved by allowing PSs to be any member of the Allied Health professions (NMC, 2018)

Communicate with your practice assessor and supervisors as to your level of experience. A plan can then be formed to allow you to maximise the learning opportunities and to identify what outcomes can be achieved during the placement period. It is important to record and clarify what your PA/PS expects from you as a nursing student. Some may want you to support the healthcare support workers to allow you to learn the fundamentals of nursing practice, and others may expect you to be able to lead a team of patients. It's important to openly discuss this early on in the placement to ensure there is no miscommunication.

Managing university placement expectations

Being a nursing student means being an ambassador of the university you are studying at. It is expected of the nursing student to adhere to the policies and guidelines set by the university and the health board they are situated in. Pay particular attention to the uniform policy, placement attendance, and how to report absences, as this will allow your university to provide additional support should it be needed. As a representative of the university, it will be expected of you to act professionally at all times, be it whilst on placement or on social media.

Managing patient's expectations

It may not be clear to people that you are a nursing student, but it is key to introduce yourself as such. People will expect the same standard of care, be it from a nursing student or a registered member of staff. Students are granted a supernumerary status, which has been mentioned earlier on in the chapter, to enable them to learn and as such focus on becoming proficient with the fundamental tasks first such as personal care and performing observations. Be open and honest about your role and take the time to get to know the patients. You may find that when you ask a patient for consent to do something you have never done before, they decline as they would prefer a more experienced staff member to perform the task. This is perfectly okay – please remember this is unlikely to be about you personally and has more to do with the patient and their past experiences.

WHO CAN YOU LEARN FROM?

The answer to that is everyone. Whilst you will spend a lot of time working alongside Registered Nurses and healthcare assistants who will all provide fundamental learning for you during your first few placements, healthcare assistants are the backbone of the direct care that patients receive and working with the healthcare assistants will be integral to developing your skills and confidence as a Registered Nurse.

Multi-discinplinary team

It's not only nursing-related staff that you can learn from, but there are also many other people whom you can gain valuable insights from. So don't be afraid to ask to spend time with other healthcare professionals too. They can give you a deeper insight into the patient journey.

NMC

THE CODE SAYS

22.3   keep your knowledge and skills up to date, taking part in appropriate and regular learning and professional development activities that aim to maintain and develop your competence and improve your performance.

CASE STUDY

Romy was on placement within cardiac rehab, which was a service run by Registered Nurses and Physiotherpaists for patients who had recently had a myocardial infarction. During this time, she spent time with the physiotherapists who were able to show her how they helped patients set realistic goals and educate patients on the benefit of exercise and healthy lifestyles post-MI.

Patients

Another group of people whom you can learn from are the patients and their families. As a nursing student, you are in a privileged position to be able to spend more time with patients than permanent staff can. Patient narratives are a very powerful tool and many are experts in their conditions and so will be able to offer you insights as to how their health condition impacts their day-to-day life.

Spoke placements

'The hub and spoke model is one approach to nursing students' practice learning, which involves a base practice placement (hub), from which the student's learning is complemented by additional activities (spokes)' (Millar, Conlon, & McGirr, 2017).

These short/satellite placements are within a specialised area connected to your practice area (hub) where you can spend some time to gain a deeper insight. For example, if you have a health visitor placement you may wish to spend some time with local charities, council-run initiatives such as parenting classes, drug and alcohol councillors, or other services you may come across which are located in the local community. These extra experiences allow you to understand the services which you can access and refer to and what their roles are.

TWEET
@ChloeCScott01

'On the district, booked time with palliative care specialist nurses - amazing! So interesting to see the other side of the palliative care plan & how decisions were made re each pt. Attended MDT meeting, getting to see how the different professions fed into overall care plan. Went for a day with the acute diabetic specialist nurse who reviewed inpatients. That was an eye opener to how poorly diabetes is managed in hospitals. It was a great opportunity for me to learn more about diabetes & how/why they would titrate doses and/or change regime.

Cardiology: had day in cath lab. Saw 37 y/o patient having STEMI & the incredible intervention of team to unblock artery & insert a stent. Weeks later saw same patient in cardiac rehab. Sadly was still engaging in adverse behaviours which could result in cardiac stent failure. I went out for the day with the Parkinson's nurse, which again was great to see the specialist advice & therapies offered to pts and carers/relatives. My advice to all students... take the opportunity to experience as much as you can as a StN! Arrange days/time with as many professionals as you can to increase knowledge/awareness. You won't get this time again'

THRIVING ON SHIFT

Turning up to placement is one thing; however, this section breaks down how to really and truly enhance the nursing student's learning experience and exposure in the clinical environment.

Looking after yourself

Being a nursing student is stressful. In order to practice safely and perform at your best, it is essential that you look after yourself. This is something that many students struggle with but burnout rates are prevalent amongst nursing students (Wei et al., 2021). Therefore, whilst it's easy to put yourself last on the priority list, it's essential that you don't.

The concept of 'self-care' is about adopting healthy lifestyle choices in order to cope with your studies, placements, and your personal life. Similar to Registered Nurses, nursing students face anxiety and stress, including the fear of the unknown in terms of knowledge or clinical skills, possibility of making mistakes, and the concept of death and dying (Admi et al., 2018). Nursing students also have stress related to their university courses, intense workloads, assignments, grades, and financial burdens (Grant-Smith and de Zwaan, 2019).

Here are some ideas of what you can do to make sure you are looking after yourself. This is only a small selection of things; the most important thing is that you do what you enjoy or what works for you.

TIP

Eat well, get enough sleep, keep hydrated, and exercise regularly. You may laugh when people say this to you and often wonder where people think you will get the time to do this. But once you start to implement it into everyday life, you will start to feel the benefits. I started to implement it into my life, and I felt better.

Practice gratitude, regularly reflect on the things you are grateful for. Now, this could be as simple as waking up in the morning or the fact that you can study nursing. But it will create a positive attitude and make you feel a lot better. A great website in line with this is Action for Happiness (https://actionforhappiness.org/). The charity's mission is to promote a happier world, through a culture that prioritises happiness and kindness. The website is packed full of useful tools, podcasts, and ways to connect with like-minded people. Alternatively, there are other platforms out there and it's up to you to find which one resonates best with you.

Lastly, in terms of self-care, it's important to make yourself familiar with the signs of stress and burnout, particularly those that may be specific to you. Burnout is the cause of unmanaged chronic stress.

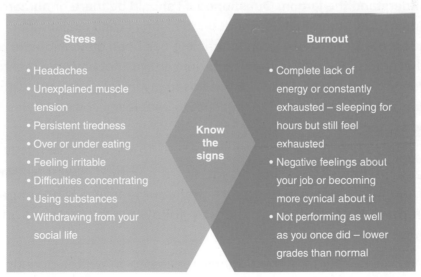

Stress

- Headaches
- Unexplained muscle tension
- Persistent tiredness
- Over or under eating
- Feeling irritable
- Difficulties concentrating
- Using substances
- Withdrawing from your social life

Know the signs

Burnout

- Complete lack of energy or constantly exhausted – sleeping for hours but still feel exhausted
- Negative feelings about your job or becoming more cynical about it
- Not performing as well as you once did – lower grades than normal

We have spoken already about where you can seek support but remember that if you have tried these things and there is no improvement, it is important you seek professional advice, such as your GP.

FEELING PART OF THE TEAM

In order to continually develop clinical skills, it is crucial that the nursing student feels supported and nurtured by the environment they are in. Inevitably, sometimes there will be setbacks but usually they can be easily resolved.

TWEET
@gunnergal4:

'The nurse in charge said to another nurse 'sorry, you're going to have to have the student'…. I was literally stood next to her, thankfully the placement got better'

TWEET
@laurielouiseB:

'Like a shaking leaf washing in, completely clueless. Handover , didn't understand the jargon. Questioned if I should be there or numerous times throughout that day. Kept on thinking , I can't ask another question. The last two years of training has been difficult due to covid challenges. Something that I experienced was not having a mentor due to shortage of staff. With this I used my initiative to work with nurses who were available that shift to enable my competencies to be signed off'

In these instances, it's important to remember that this can still be turned into a positive to ensure that your learning is not impacted. It is important to seek guidance by following the process in your documentation.

However, in positive contrast, many replies to a Twitter question had many stating that they were made to feel welcome.

TWEET

@HannahBnurse03:

'I was nervous but loved it. I remember the nurse I was working with went and put my name on the nurse board next to hers and made me feel part of the team'

TWEET

@Rachela98176019:

'My first placement I was so petrified but within the first hour of being there I was totally took under their wing and to this day I have remained friends with some of the nurses. They put so much time and effort into teaching me and had shown me so much trust'

TWEET

@RNA_Ni_:

'My first placement was with@Worksopnurses and from day one I was made to feel welcome and part of the team. I was very lucky to have such a great start to my course ☺'

TWEET

@HeatherKchn:

'You do hear horror stories but the best part about of being a student nurse is getting to feel like a nurse and I couldn't have asked for a better experience on my 1st placement. The team made me feel welcome and included me in everything and I got wonderful feedback'

TWEET

@LawrenceReb:

'I have to say it was an incredible experience and can only describe being in the position of being able to sit with and hold the hand of a dying patient the biggest honour of my life'

It's important that you use your initiative while on placement. For example, during the handover you may hear about a procedure that a patient is due to have that you have never seen be performed, so you could ask to observe or assist whoever is doing it. This shows you are enthusiastic and keen to learn.

Another key, but simple, thing to do, is to just muck in and lend a helping hand when things are busy. This will show you are a team player.

Lastly, 'there is no such thing as a stupid question', so please ask questions. The world of nursing is a never-ending learning journey, and as a nursing student this is very much the beginning. If the answer will benefit your learning, then don't be afraid to ask, and in addition it may make the other person reflect on why they do things the way they do. It's essential to try to be as diplomatic as possible and be more curious than interrogatory.

The NMC advocates that Registsered Nurses and students practice within their own sphere of competency. As a student it is not expected that you will know everything as soon as you begin and it's good practice to try and understand the reasons why procedures are carried out.

As you can see, there are plenty of ways to make the most of your placement time; you just need to be focused and take an active role in your learning. Remember, communication is key, so you need to keep reminding people what you want to learn.

COMMUNICATION

It can be a nerve-wracking experience communicating with colleagues, relatives, or anybody in general who could potentially ask you a question you have no idea how to answer in your nursing infancy. However, it is vital to learn to communicate effectively.

NMC | THE CODE SAYS

7.1 use terms that people in your care, colleagues and the public can understand

NMC | THE CODE SAYS

8.2 maintain effective communication with colleagues

Why is it a struggle though when communication tools are taught as part of the programme? The answer could be simply that confidence is lacking, as discussed by Skarbaliene, Skarbalius, and Gedrine (2019), especially if this is your first foray into the healthcare world. It takes time to become comfortable in your new environment, and it's not uncommon to see students almost glued to their PA/PS's at the beginning of their placement experience.

CASE STUDY

Krishna is a nursing student and is on placement at an elderly care ward. During one shift towards the end of a shift all the ward staff are handing over and there is a huddle of nursing students converging on the nurse's station when the ward phone starts ringing. The panic sets in and everyone just looks at each other blankly, hoping someone else will commit to answering the call. The longer it rings, the more the pressure builds. Krishna is unsure of what to do and feels that they don't have enough experience or knowledge to pick up the phone and potentially have to deal with something unfamiliar to them.

> ✏️ **What would you do if faced with a situation similar to Krishna's?**
>
> _____
>
> _____
>
> _____
>
> _____
>
> _____
>
> _____

In a corresponding Twitter poll, nearly 38% of nursing students claimed that during their first year, they would run for the hills rather than talk to the person on the other end due to a lack of confidence.

It is important to recognise that you aren't expected to know everything. If you are asked something which you don't know, it is okay to say you will find out or get someone who does know. This is much better than giving wrong information that could cause potential harm to patients.

Communication is something humans often do without thinking. Working in a healthcare environment means it's important to be mindful of how information is conveyed, be it verbally, in written notes, or when data is sent electronically.

NMC THE CODE SAYS

1: Treat people as individuals and uphold their dignity.

NMC THE CODE SAYS

5: Respect people's right to privacy and confidentiality.

For instance, imagine you are involved in a handover on your placement ward and the information is being given to you in a bay full of other patients. Do you think this would be a breach of the patient's privacy? How would it make you feel if that were you?

Whenever information is transmitted to other staff or relatives it is governed by the Human Rights Act, the Data Protection Act, and the Caldicott Principles, which means only relevant and necessary information should be relayed in a secure manner. The Caldicott Principles are listed below:

Principle 1: Justify the purpose(s) for using confidential information
Principle 2: Use confidential information only when it is necessary
Principle 3: Use the minimum necessary confidential information
Principle 4: Access to confidential information should be on a strict need-to-know basis
Principle 5: Everyone with access to confidential information should be aware of their responsibilities
Principle 6: Comply with the law
Principle 7: The duty to share information for individual care is as important as the duty to protect patient confidentiality
Principle 8: Inform patients and service users about how their confidential information is used

Documentation and paperwork

When you first encounter the patient notes, they may seem as thick as the bible, with the chances of finding the right section and deciphering the handwriting being probably less than winning the lottery. They are generally a mixture of nursing care plans and notes, doctors' notes, relevant treatment information, and any other relevant patient history. The more acquainted you become with patient notes, the easier your nursing journey will be.

The daily ritual of documenting a patient's notes in one shared by Registered Nurses worldwide. This is done to hand over information and to keep the patients and our colleagues safe. The old adage of 'If you didn't write it, it didn't happen' can come sharply into focus if an incident occurs, the patient's health deteriorates, or treatment is delayed due to an accurate and timely handover not occurring (Elliott, 2022).

NMC

THE CODE SAYS

10.3 complete records accurately and without any falsification, taking immediate and appropriate action if you become aware that someone has not kept to these requirements

Depending on your placement area you will need to cover a core set of care plans, such as the skin bundle, ongoing treatment, nutritional intake, and any other developments that are vital to the patient's ongoing care planning. Your local Health Trust will invariably have slight changes in the documentation that is required to be completed; however, a useful guide of how patient notes should be maintained can be simplified into:

DOCUMENTATION	
DO	**DON'T**
• Write legibly and in black pen	• Abbreviate
• Take your time	• Cover mistakes with Tipp-Ex
• Put a line through and initial any mistakes	• Duplicate the previous day's notes
• Be precise and accurate	• Be ambiguous or use jargon
• Cite facts and evidence	• Over-complicate the entry
• Use appropriate language	• Speculate
• Be professional	
• Remain objective	

One of the most important relationships that you'll make while on placement is with your practice assessor/supervisor, so it's important to take the time to build an effective and professional working relationship. Unfortunately, this relationship doesn't always work. Sometimes, staff can be conflicted over their duty to you as a student and the competing duty to patients, leaving them feeling frustrated. It's important to remember that this isn't personal. Also, we are human, and we don't get along with everyone – it may be that you simply have a clash of personalities. That is okay, but it is crucial that you remain professional. However, if you feel that you are being treated unprofessionally, please consider keeping written evidence of what happened and when so that you can inform your university and ask for their help. It could be down to poor supervision, and by reporting it, you are ensuring that future students aren't adversely affected.

Creating professional boundaries

Peternelj-Taylor (2002) defines professional boundaries as the limitations that the Registered Nurse can operate within in order to deliver effective care. Furthermore, it is a requirement, and expectation, of the Registered Nurse to facilitate a professional partnership with the patient where there are clearly defined boundaries and the relationship should not be deemed as friendship (NMC, 2018; Valente, 2017). Professional boundaries seek to ensure that the nurse-patient relationship is safe and respectful and maintains a professional distance between Registered Nurse and patient with care servicing the patient, not the Registered Nurse (Mendes, 2017; Valente, 2017).

From the beginning of the relationship, it is the role of the Registered Nurse to educate and enforce the limitations of the relationship concerning the physical, emotional, sexual, and social limits; however, as the relationship is fluid, these boundaries must be continually reassessed for their relevance (McCormack and McCance, 2017; Peternelj-Taylor, 2002). Any violation of the boundaries, from either the Registered Nurse or the patient, may erode trust, harm the patient, diminish the therapeutic relationship, and result in disciplinary action for the Registered Nurse (NMC, 2018; Valente, 2017).

There are two types of boundary violations: professional and ethical. Professional violations include sexual and non-sexual misconduct, such as favouritism, giving or receiving of gifts, sexual touching, and over-familiarity (Chiarella and Adrian, 2014; Manfrin-Ledet, Porche, and Eymard, 2015). Ethical violations relate to the competency and integrity of the Registered Nurse, such as fraudulent nursing documentation, violation of the Registered Nurses professional duty of candour, and physically, or emotionally, neglecting the patient (NMC, 2018).

Emotional intelligence is crucial for the Registered Nurse as it allows them to observe their emotions and reflect when they feel the strains of their profession, seeking peer support when appropriate. Creating a boundary and achieving a work-life balance is important not only in the interest of the patient but also to prevent burnout of the Registered Nurse, allowing them to work effectively and keep any concerns about the patient restricted to when they are working. Since the early 2000s, Registered Nurses are increasingly using social media for professional purposes in their private and professional lives (Stott, 2015); therefore, it is important that a balance is found between the benefits associated with social media and the potential for violating professional boundaries. As it is the duty of the Registered Nurse to maintain and safeguard the privacy of the patients, Registered Nurses must act with caution in relation to social media, in order not to devalue the trust that may have been created within the therapeutic relationship through a breach of confidentiality. It is essential that the Registered Nurse refuses any invitations from patients to connect via social media, therefore extending the professional relationship into a personal context.

CASE STUDY

Eddie was an enthusiastic student who wanted to make the most of his time at university. He would often say 'yes' to every extra-curricular opportunity that came his way or when friends and family wanted to spend time with him – even after a long and challenging day. By the end of his 2nd year at university, he was exhausted. He couldn't focus on any one task and he couldn't get to sleep because his mind was whirring. His friends and family noticed that he had lost his sparkle and his nursing peers saw that he wasn't as enthusiastic as he once was.

In this case study, it is clear that Eddie spread himself too thinly. Whilst it is important to develop your skills, it is important to focus on the activities that bring you energy. Spending time with family and friends is important but it would be helpful if you explained to them the expectations and demands of the course so that they understand that you may not be around as much as you once were.

Feedback

Providing feedback to the nursing student is a core element of PS and should be provided by the practice assessor and supervisors, as set out by the NMC (2018).

NMC

THE CODE SAYS

3.3 support and supervise students, providing feedback on their progress towards, and achievement of, proficiencies and skills

Throughout the placement, via a series of progression point interviews the nursing student will be assessed and this will include feedback. Constructive feedback is encouraged as it can aid in development and highlight areas of practice which may need further attention.

Feedback should be a two-way interaction with the practice assessor receiving a report from the supervisor but also asking the student to evaluate their own performance (NMC, 2018). A crucial part of providing feedback is including relevant observations on the student's conduct, proficiency, and achievement to the student's record(s) of achievement (NMC, 2018). These observations may include the remarks of anyone else who has taken an active part in the student's teaching (NMC, 2018).

A crucial part of providing feedback is including relevant observations on the student's conduct, proficiency, and achievement to the student's record(s) of achievement (NMC, 2018). These observations may include the remarks of anyone else who has taken an active part in the student's teaching (NMC, 2018).

POST-PLACEMENT (WELL DONE!!!)

Once you have finished your day, you may just want to get home and crawl into bed. But it's always worth thinking about your day. Perhaps ask yourself the following questions:

What went well?
What could you have done differently?
What did you learn?
What do you need to learn?

This will allow your learning to progress but also think about situations you may have done differently. You may also want to consider the going home checklist.

Going home checklist
☑ Take a moment to think about today.
☑ Acknowledge one thing that was difficult during your working day – let it go.
☑ Consider three things that went well.
☑ Check on your colleagues before you leave – are they OK?
☑ Are you OK? Your senior team are here to support you.
☑ Now switch your attention to home – rest and recharge.

REFLECTION: LEARNING FROM ACTIONS

'Observation tells us fact, reflection the meaning of the fact'

– Florence Nightingale

Once you have completed the set number of hours for that placement, there is still a bit more you need to do before you can fully relax. Reflection is intrinsic to our learning and helps develop our competence. The use of reflection is a highly beneficial method for Registered Nurses to explore and examine themselves, their perspectives, attributes, experiences, actions, and interactions to give insight into becoming more competent practitioners (Anderson, 2019; Ellis, 2017). Critical reflection is more than thinking; it aims to develop understanding in a structured, focused, and conscious way (Payne, 2015). Used effectively, it anchors experiential learning to make sense of a situation at a specific point in time by analysing and critiquing the who, what, why, when, and how of the event (Driscoll, 2007; Gibbs, 1988; Johns, 2013).

Using a reflective model is useful for those who are new to reflection as it provides a structured formula which provides a starting point and gives the reflection direction to produce stronger, more focused critical reflection (Jansen and Hanssen, 2017; van Bruchem-Visser et al., 2020). There are many reflective models available that will act as a framework to help you. Here are a few to look up:

- Driscoll Model of Reflection: perhaps one of the simplest models and stems from three questions: What? So What? Now What?
- Gibbs' Reflective Cycle: one of the most commonly used reflective cycles in nursing. It looks at experiences allowing learning and planning from things that either did or didn't go well.
- Johns Model of Reflection: this encourages you to look at the experience from a range of standpoints and to consider the learner's actions not only on other people 'Looking outwards' but also on themselves 'looking inwards'.
- Rolfe's Model: this model considers what happened, the impact of the event, and the consequences for the future.

Placements provide ample opportunities for reflection, but we do become very task focused on placement and can find ourselves just wanting to pass or get our competencies signed off. However, we need to deepen our thinking; the purpose of reflection is to move forward and grow. It can help you make sense of the situations that you find yourself in.

 TIP

Keeping a reflective journal is useful as it can help to clarify your values, affirm your strengths, and identify your learning needs – it will also be good practice to move forward with for when you are a Registered Nurse and need to revalidate.

TWEET

@nursescorneruk1:

'Oh yes, always makes my revalidation easy. Reflective practice is an important part of your professional development. This is helped me to identify my strengths and areas of improvement'

'I keep one after each placement, it helps to show me what I've learned and areas I should focus on in my next placement to ensure my knowledge and skills keep growing'

–Zoe Dixon, nursing student

TROUBLESHOOTING

What to do if you haven't heard about your placement location from university

If the countdown to your placement is approaching quickly and you haven't heard from the placement team at your university then it would be advisable to send them a polite email. Remember that you are expected to demonstrate professionalism when communicating with colleagues and the chances are they are working hard to secure you a position and are waiting for a response from the clinical area.

What to do if you have concerns with your practice assessor or practice supervisor

Unfortunately, not every placement will be your favourite placement and some students will have concerns involving their practice assessor, if learning requirements are not being met, or if an incident occurs. If things aren't going to plan, don't panic! Share the problem through the proper channels and remember to remain professional. If you feel you can't talk to your practice assessor or supervisor, contact your placements team, or even your academic tutor in university who will give you the name of the designated staff member who will be the placement facilitator for the area. Raising concerns needs to be done in the right way. Your university should have a policy in place to guide you through this process.

Why is it important to be able to communicate effectively

Sometimes, things don't always go to plan, and we may encounter problems along the way. Normally you find when problems occur, it's usually down to lack of communication. Placement can often be a busy time and you may struggle to discuss any external factors with your practice assessor or supervisor. You may feel embarrassed, or you don't want to bother them while they are busy. But it's vital that you do.

'It can be advantageous to let the placement area know if there are certain times of the week that you simply cannot work. For instance, I have had instances where I have had no child care and it is not possible to book breakfast or after school clubs at short notice. By being upfront (politely and tactfully) I found it easier to get my rota in advance. I usually discussed this with my practice assessor at the start but also found it was good to inform the area once I had found out my placement as it gives them a heads up of who to allocate you to. Most ward managers are fine and understand you have commitments outside the course'.

– Simon James, Community Registered Nurse

What to deal with the physical demands of placement

Something nursing students may face while on placement is tiredness. You might not deem this as a 'problem', but it's definitely a challenge that should be considered. You may not be used to 12-hour shifts, and they can be physically and emotionally tiring. You could find that your body aches or you may not be used to getting up so early. You may find it difficult to sleep during the day after a night shift leaving you exhausted. It's important that you listen to your body, try not to do lots of 12-hour shifts in a row (many universities advocate not to work three long shifts in a row) and make sure you take time out for yourself, which is easier said than done!

What to do if you are feeling isolated

Something that isn't spoken about enough is the isolation some nursing students face while on placement. As mentioned previously, while you are on theory block at university, you have the structure of knowing where you are going to be and you have the support from your peers (granted, online learning can make this a little more challenging). However, while on placement, you may find that you are the only one there from your cohort, or you may be the only student, which can result in you feeling isolated. As a result of working shifts, it can be difficult to arrange a time to meet your peers that works for everyone. It's encouraged to 'find your tribe' and set up a group chat so you can at least keep in contact with them – remember to be professional, as even private groups can still get you into trouble. All it takes is for someone to misconstrue what you have said, then screenshot it and send it to uni – remember to familiarise yourself with the NMC's social media guidance.

NMC

THE CODE SAYS

20.10 use all forms of spoken, written and digital communication (including social media and networking sites) responsibly, respecting the right to privacy of others at all times

Where to get support?

If you have raised an issue, it's important to know where support can be accessed. It has already been mentioned that your practice assessor and supervisor are your main sources of support while on placement, so they should be your first point of contact.

- Your peers. They are on this journey with you and understand what the challenges are. Speak to them if you need some extra support – you never know, they may have lived experience of what you are going through and may be able to offer some handy advice.

- Your academic advisor – if you feel your learning is being compromised, it's advisable to reach out and ask for help so that your progression isn't impacted.
- University support services. Universities have wonderful services to really help students.
- Your friends and family – they may not understand the challenges you are facing but they do know you and they will want to help in whatever way they can.
- Hospital chaplain – it's important to remember that you may encounter things that you have never experienced before, such as death and dying, so you can always contact them if you feel you need some holistic or spiritual support.

CONCLUSION

Placements are an exciting part of being a nursing student, but they can also be anxiety provoking. In this chapter, we have taken you through the journey of your nursing placement, from how to prepare to what to expect and how to reflect.

It is essential to remember that this journey is unique to you, but you aren't alone. There are plenty of places to seek support to help you make the most of it. But the most important piece of advice we can give you is to try your best to enjoy it – even on the hardest of days.

'Happiness can be found, even in the darkest of times, if one only remembers to turn on the light'.

– Dumbledore

Now, that you have finished this chapter. Make some notes on what you have learned.

REFERENCES

Admi, H., Moshe-Eilon, Y., Sharon, D. and Mann, M., 2018. Nursing students' stress and satisfaction in clinical practice along different stages: A cross-sectional study. *Nurse Education Today*, 68, pp. 86–92.

Anderson, B., 2019. Reflecting on the communication process in health care. Part 1: Clinical practice-breaking bad news. *British Journal of Nursing*, [online] 28(13), pp. 858–863. Available at: <https://www-magonlinelibrary-com.gcu.idm.oclc.org/doi/abs/10.12968/bjon.2019.28.13.858> [Accessed 14 Nov. 2021].

Chiarella, M. and Adrian, A., 2014. Boundary violations, gender and the nature of nursing work. *Nursing Ethics*, [online] 21(3), pp. 267–277. Available at: <https://journals-sagepub-com.gcu.idm.oclc.org/doi/full/10.1177/0969733013493214> [Accessed 24 Feb. 2022].

Driscoll, J., 2007. *Practising Clinical Supervision: A Reflective Approach for Healthcare Professionals*. 2nd ed. Edinburgh: Elsevier.

Elliott, N., 2022. Get on top of your record-keeping skills. *Nursing Standard*, [online] 37(2), pp. 41–42. Available at: <https://journals.rcni.com/doi/10.7748/ns.37.2.41.s19> [Accessed 14 Feb. 2022].

Ellis, N., 2017. Decision making in practice: Influences, management and reflection. *British Journal of Nursing*, [online] 26(2), pp. 109–112. Available at: <https://www-magonlinelibrary-com.gcu.idm.oclc.org/doi/abs/10.12968/bjon.2017.26.2.109> [Accessed 15 Nov. 2021].

El-Sharkawy, A.M., Bragg, D., Watson, P., Neal, K., Sahota, O., Maughan, R.J. and Lobo, D.N., 2016. Hydration amongst nurses and doctors on-call (the HANDS on prospective cohort study). *Clinical Nutrition*, 35(4), pp. 935–942.

Gibbs, G., 1988. *Learning by Doing: A Guide to Teaching and Learning Methods*. London: Further Education Unit.

Granger, K., 2013. Healthcare staff must properly introduce themselves to patients. *BMJ*, [online]. Available at: <https://www-bmj-com.gcu.idm.oclc.org/content/347/bmj.f5833> [Accessed 20 Feb. 2022].

Grant-Smith, D. and de Zwaan, L., 2019. Don't spend, eat less, save more: Responses to the financial stress experienced by nursing students during unpaid clinical placements. *Nurse Education in Practice*, 35, pp. 1–6.

Jansen, T.L. and Hanssen, I., 2017. Patient participation: Causing moral stress in psychiatric nursing? *Scandinavian Journal of Caring Sciences*, [online] 31(2), pp. 388–394. Available at: <https://onlinelibrary-wiley-com.gcu.idm.oclc.org/doi/full/10.1111/scs.12358> [Accessed 4 Jan. 2022].

Johns, C., 2013. *Becoming a Reflective Practitioner*. [online] Wiley-Blackwell. Available at: <https://www.dawsonera.com:443/abstract/9781118492291> [Accessed 14 Nov. 2021].

Manfrin-Ledet, L., Porche, D.J. and Eymard, A.S., 2015. Professional boundary violations: A literature review. *Home Healthcare Now*, 33(6), pp. 326–332.

Mansel, B., & Einion, A. (2019). 'It's the relationship you develop with them': emotional intelligence in nurse leadership. A qualitative study. British journal of nursing, 28 21, 1400–1408. DOI:10.12968/bjon.2019.28.21.1400

McCormack, B. and McCance, T., 2017. *Person-Centred Nursing: Theory and Practice.* 2nd ed. Chichester: Wiley-Blackwell.

Mendes, A., 2017. Nursing care and maintaining professional boundaries. *British Journal of Community Nursing*, [online] 22(8), pp. 407–408. Available at: <https://www-magonlinelibrary-com.gcu.idm.oclc.org/doi/abs/10.12968/bjcn.2017.22.8.407> [Accessed 24 Feb. 2022].

Millar L, Conlon M, McGirr D. Students' perspectives of using the hub and spoke model to support and develop learning in practice. Nurs Stand. 2017;32(9):41-49. doi:10.7748/ns.2017.e10389

NHS Employers, 2020. *Uniforms and Workwear: Guidance for NHS Employers.* [online] Available at: <https://www.england.nhs.uk/wp-content/uploads/2020/04/Uniforms-and-Workwear-Guidance-2-April-2020.pdf> [Accessed 3 May 2022].

Nursing and Midwifery Council, 2018a. *The Code for Nurses and Midwives.* [online] Available at: <https://www.nmc.org.uk/standards/code/read-the-code-online/> [Accessed 15 Nov. 2021].

Nursing and Midwifery Council, 2018b. *Future Nurse: Standards of Proficiency for Registered Nurses.* [online] Available at: <https://www.nmc.org.uk/globalassets/sitedocuments/standards-of-proficiency/nurses/future-nurse-proficiencies.pdf> [Accessed 3 Jan. 2022].

Nursing and Midwifery Council, 2018c. *Future Nurse: Standards of Proficiency for Registered Nurses: What Do Practice Assessors Do?* [online] Available at: <https://www.nmc.org.uk/supporting-information-on-standards-for-student-supervision-and-assessment/practice-assessment/what-do-practice-assessors-do/> [Accessed 3 Jan. 2022].

Payne, M., 2015. A Beginner's Guide to Critical Thinking and Writing in Health and Social Care, 2nd edn. *British Journal of Social Work*, 45(7), pp. 2229–2231.

Peternelj-Taylor, C., 2002. Professional boundaries: A matter of therapeutic integrity. *Journal of Psychosocial Nursing and Mental Health Services*, 40(4), pp. 23–29.

Royal College of Nursing, 2021. Healthy Workplace, Healthy You. Available at: <https://www.rcn.org.uk/healthy-workplace/healthy-you/time-and-space> [Accessed 3 May 2022].

Skarbaliene, A., Skarbalius, E. and Gedrime, L., 2019. Effective communication in the healthcare settings: are the graduates ready for it? doi:10.30924/mjcmi.24.si.9

Stott, I., 2015. Social media in the workplace: approach with caution. *Nursing and Residential Care,* 17(9), pp. 519–521. Available at: <https://doi.org/10.12968/nrec.2015.17.9.519>.

UK Government, 1998. Human Rights Act 1998. Available at: <https://www.legislation.gov.uk/ukpga/1998/42/contents> [Accessed 21 Feb. 2022].

UK Government, 2020. The Caldicott Principles. Available at: <https://www.gov.uk/government/publications/the-caldicott-principles> [Accessed 14 March 2022].

Valente, S.M., 2017. Managing professional and nurse–patient relationship boundaries in mental health. *Journal of Psychosocial Nursing and Mental Health Services*, 55(1), pp. 45–51.

van Bruchem-Visser, R.L., van Dijk, G., de Beaufort, I. and Mattace-Raso, F., 2020. Ethical frameworks for complex medical decision making in older patients: A narrative review. *Archives of Gerontology and Geriatrics*, 90, p. 104160. DOI: 10.1016/j.archger.2020.104160 [Accessed 14 Nov. 2021].

Watt, E., Murphy, M., MacDonald, L., Pascoe, E., Storen, H. and Scanlon, A., 2016. An evaluation of a structured learning program as a component of the clinical practicum in undergraduate nurse education: A repeated measures analysis. *Nurse Education Today*, 36, pp. 172–177.

Wei, H., Dorn, A., Hutto, H., Corbett, R.W., Haberstroh, A. and Larson, K., 2021. Impacts of nursing student burnout on psychological well-being and academic achievement. *Journal of Nursing Education*, 60(7), pp. 369–376.

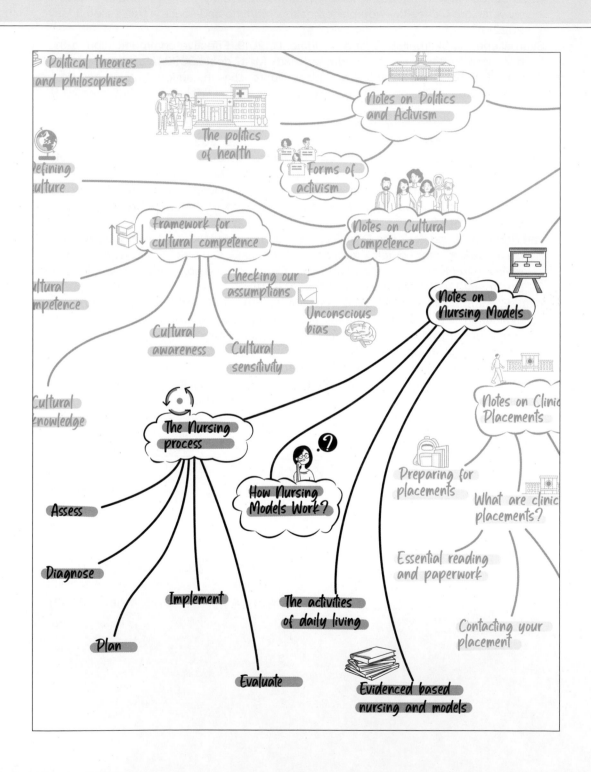

NOTES ON NURSING MODELS

Sally Wilson (She/Her)

INTRODUCTION

'The unique function of the nurse is to assist the individual, sick or well, in the performance of those activities contributing to the health or its recovery (or to a peaceful death) that he would perform unaided if he had the necessary strength, will or knowledge'.

— Virginia Henderson

In an increasingly complex world, there are a growing number of ways in which we can fulfil our nursing duties. To achieve this there are a variety of skills and tools at our disposal. We just need to learn which ones we need at any given time. This in itself is a skill nursing students need to master — which can be more challenging than learning practical nursing skills and techniques!

For each clinical nursing skill there is a process behind it, with a rationale and several clinical decision points which guide Registered Nurses in how to respond (Perry, Potter, and Ostendorf 2014). It is the combination of a number of nursing skills and processes which forms part of a nursing model — therefore a model can be described as a way of representing the reality of nursing (Murphy, Williams, and Pridmore 2010).

Some nursing models to explore include:

- Activities of living — Roper, Logan, and Tierney (1990)
- Self care model — Orem (1991)

- The Moulster and Griffiths learning and disability nursing model – Moulster and Griffith (2012)
- Peplau's Theory (1988)
- Casey's Model of Nursing (1988)

Nursing models can initially be a tricky concept to get to grips with as a nursing student but ultimately, they can support and improve nursing practice, so they are definitely something worth understanding.

THE BENEFITS OF NURSING MODELS

Developing models to shape the direction of modern nursing is something which has been at the forefront of nursing leadership since the 1980s (Pearson, Vaughan, and Fitzgerald 2005).

The use of a model in the development of nursing documentation especially is important to provide a comprehensive and holistic assessment and care planning tool. A nursing model can support Registered Nurses to develop competence in the assessment and delivery of clinical skills providing a framework on which to practice. Models can also give nursing students real confidence that they are meeting all their patients' needs.

TWEET

@Amy_5haw:

'I think models help us to frame things in a way that help us to add value #valuebasedhealthcare@WeNurses it's important we have a framework so that we can cover all ground that requires covering to meet someone's needs'

The aim and benefit of a nursing model is primarily to describe and enable the nursing process.

According to Toney-Butler and Thayer (2022), the nursing process has five sequential stages which are (Fig 6.1):

- Assessment
- Diagnosis
- Planning

- Implementation
- Evaluation.

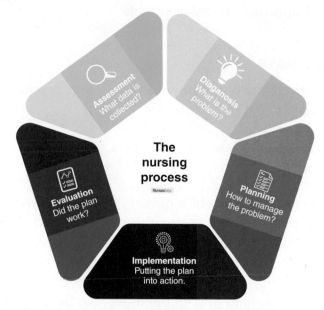

Figure 6.1   The Nursing Process. (Wayne G (2022) The Nursing Process: A comprehensive guide Nurseslabs Available at https://nurseslabs.com/ nursing-process/ (last accessed 23/9/22).

For nursing students, and newly Registered Nurses, navigating the five stages of the nursing process can be daunting and has a seemingly endless list of components to remember, assess, and act on.

Nursing is a process which is diverse and complex in nature and as such it requires careful consideration at each stage:

Assessment

Registered Nurses must consider the assessment process, which assessment tools to use and the application of the assessment findings to the planning of care. There are a myriad of assessment tools available to support patient care, but they are all derived from a nursing model. The assessments will provide data which informs the other stages within the process; some of the assessment process involves obtaining a clinical history from the patient, for example, or taking a set of observations such as temperature, pulse, blood pressure, etc. Assessment can be complex and time consuming, and often there are several variables which need to be considered. Using a nursing model can help to shape the assessment process and discussions with the patient while still ensuring a holistic approach to assessment.

> **NMC**
>
> ### THE CODE SAYS
>
> 3 **Make sure that people's physical, social and psychological needs are assessed and responded to**

Diagnosis

This involves the formulation of a nursing diagnosis, which differs from a medical diagnosis in that it states the nursing need and informs the care plan and clinical decision making. Toney-Butler and Thayer (2022) state this element of the nursing process must consider a person's basic physiological needs, for example, the need for nutrition, hydration, and toileting. Security and safety must also be considered – these are all stages within Maslow's hierarchy of needs.

Planning

This stage involves using the tool chosen to decide and document how care will be delivered, what will be recorded, and when it will be reviewed. This part of the process enables goal setting and measurable outcomes for the patient aimed to improve their physiological status or promote comfort care. It is important to consider how goals are set within individualised care planning and hence the SMART algorithm can be used, Goals should be:

1. Specific
2. Measurable or Meaningful
3. Attainable or Action-Oriented
4. Realistic or Results-Oriented
5. Timely or Time-Oriented

Implementation

The Registered Nurse ensures that the care plan is delivered to the patient; this can be achieved through direct patient intervention, referral to other healthcare practitioners, or liaison with members of the multi-disciplinary team.

Evaluation

Registered Nurses consider what worked well, and what, if anything, requires changing to ensure patient needs are met, goals are achieved, and the patient is making progress aligned with their care plans. Once care is delivered, Registered Nurses must consider if it was effective in achieving the right outcomes for their patient, and if it has not achieved what was intended, what can be changed.

Nursing models aim to break down the nursing process into defined areas with identified skill sets attached to them. Breaking down the process makes the model easy to follow and promotes a systematic approach to assessment, treatment, and care delivery.

Nursing models enable Registered Nurses to:

- Assess the people we care for
- Plan care
- Have a clear process to underpin a task or skill, making it much easier to accomplish as the steps to attainment are within the process
- Evaluate care
- Ensure that we have taken a holistic approach to care

HOW DO MODELS WORK?

As discussed, nursing models provide a framework for the nursing process, with defined parameters for the assessment, planning, implementation, and evaluation of nursing care. In addition to this nursing models can encourage Registered Nurses and nursing students to plan effective care, identify when the plans aren't working, and make changes to these plans when improvement isn't achieved.

The use of a model ensures we are considering every aspect of nursing care we need to and therefore Registered Nurses are enabled in planning and delivering effective holistic care. Models help Registered Nurses to ensure that they are not missing any element of the care process. McKenna, Pajinkihar, and Murphy (2014) state that nursing is theory in action, as behind every nursing act there is a theory which underpins it.

If a Registered Nurse is changing a surgical dressing, the practical process of removal and replacement of a dressing is underpinned by the theory of using an aseptic technique to prevent infection. Although some Registered Nurses may argue that nursing is essentially a series of practical clinical skills, it's important to remember that there is a theoretical evidence base behind each skill. In the same way that infection prevention evidence underpins surgical dressing application nursing models provide the theoretical evidence base to assess, diagnose, plan, implement, and evaluate care.

THE ACTIVITIES OF DAILY LIVING

One of the most recognisable nursing models in the UK was designed by Roper, Logan, and Tierney who were Registered Nurses working in Scotland in the 1970s and 1980s. They based their model on 12 activities of daily living; this followed from the work of the American nurse Virginia Henderson whose theory focused on increasing and/or maintaining independence. The activities of daily living (ADLs) model married theory to practice and encourages Registered Nurses to understand why the ADLs improved patient outcomes and health needs. The ADLs, according to Roper, Logan, and Tierney, are:

- Maintaining a safe environment
- Communication
- Breathing
- Eating and drinking
- Eliminating
- Personal cleaning and dressing
- Controlling body temperature
- Mobilising
- Working and playing
- Expressing sexuality
- Sleeping
- Dying

Roper, Logan, and Tierney (2000) provide an in-depth exploration of their nursing model and the theory behind it, and this resonates with contemporary nursing, which endorses being evidence based on theory.

> 'The fundamentals of care include, but are not limited to, nutrition, hydration, bladder and bowel care, physical handling and making sure that those receiving care are kept in clean and hygienic conditions. It includes making sure that those receiving care have adequate access to nutrition and hydration, and making sure that you provide help to those who are not able to feed themselves or drink fluid unaided'.

> **– Florence Nightingale.**

The ADLs are fundamentally used as an indicator of a person's independence and functioning and form a key part of the nursing assessment. Registered Nurses are in a unique position in that they are often the first professional to observe when a person's functionality has changed due to the level of support they need. Assessments that include ADLs can help to identify both deterioration and improvement in a person's functioning which in turn can support longer-term care planning, safe discharge from acute services, and assessment for a package of care or placement if required. A person's inability to complete essential ADLs can lead to unsafe living conditions which in turn can increase risk of emergency admissions and the need to access urgent care settings (Edemekong et al. 2017). Although the ADLs were first identified over 70 years ago, they remain a valid marker of patient status and are still used in nursing practice.

According to Edemekong et al. (2017) the assessment of ADLs remains a vital component of routine patient assessment and the delivery of nursing care. This supports the identification of a patient's functional status which can indicate:

- medium- to long-term care needs,
- the requirement for further rehabilitation,
- additional support at home to maintain safety.

For example, we know patient falls are linked with increased mortality rates in older people (Ambrose, Geet, and Hausdorff 2013), and an assessment of mobility can support care planning which can mitigate the risk of people falling. Specific assessments regarding balance, gait, pace, polypharmacy, and any history of previous falls can all be used to identify current and future risk of falls according to Ambrose, Geet, and Hausdorff (2013). The prevention of falls through care interventions can be achieved in a variety of ways, such as wearing safer, properly fitted footwear and the use of mobility aids (like grab sticks or Zimmer frames etc.). The value of the ADLs and a nursing model that uses and supports the ADLs can therefore be measured by patient outcomes. In the example above this is readmission rates to an acute hospital for a patient with a known history of falls. If the care plan and interventions are successful then the admission rates for that patient should decrease, also reducing the risk of serious injury.

CASE STUDY

Doris was 86 when she was admitted to hospital after a fall. Her son provided a recent history as Doris has advancing dementia and was unable to tell the staff in the ED what had happened to her. Doris's son expressed concern about her managing at home and told staff in ED that she had been found in the street by neighbours late at night with no shoes on. Doris was admitted to the care of the elderly ward and staff started working on her nursing admission and care planning paperwork.

Doris was a secretary working in a large company. She was used to being busy and often visited other departments to help out. In her spare time she enjoyed gardening and had an allotment for many years. Doris married Frank in 1962 and they had 3 children, and she has 12 grandchildren who all live locally.

Doris is assessed as lacking the capacity to make decisions about her care and treatment. She seems much more settled when she is able to move around; she is at times non-compliant with treatment including the use of mobility aids, without which she remains at high

CASE STUDY—cont'd

risk of falls. She has tolerated the use of non-slip socks on the ward area. Doris has been assessed as being unable to make herself a hot drink, and she has shown poor functional skills in washing and dressing.

With Doris to have a package of care during the day, the family believe it is in her best interests to return to her own home, which is a single-storey bungalow, but they agree with the assessment findings that Doris needs additional support and safety planning. The occupational therapist and falls specialist feel Doris would benefit from the gas being turned off so she can't accidentally leave the oven or fire on, a falls mat by her bed and armchair, and an alarm on her front door which will alert when Doris leaves the house. Doris is also assessed as needing two care calls a day to support with personal hygiene and meal preparation.

Doris is readmitted 9 days after discharge having had a fall in her garden.

What do you think needs to be reviewed within Doris's existing care plan and how could a nursing model support this?

_____

_____

_____

_____

_____

_____

_____

The case study highlights that Doris may benefit from a full nursing assessment that assesses all of the ADLs; using Roper, Logan, and Tierney's model some of the following questions may need to be asked:

- Maintaining a safe environment – Doris is at high risk of falls; how can the team support Doris to move safely? Things like footwear, foot health, the physical environment, and how other aids (e.g. handrails) may support her.
- Communication – Doris has been identified as lacking the capacity to make decisions around her care and treatment but what does she understand and how can nursing staff support Doris to communicate?
- Breathing – Does Doris have any underlying infections? Does she have any past medical history around breathing that may affect her cognition or ability to mobilise?
- Eating and drinking – Why is Doris turning on the gas? Is she hungry or thirsty? If so, how can nursing staff support Doris to prepare food and drink independently?
- Eliminating – Is Doris able to mobilise safely enough to get to the toilet? What can be done to support her? Is Doris at risk of constipation or a urinary tract infection and if so, does this have the potential to cause any confusion with Doris?
- Personal cleaning and dressing – What support does Doris need to wash and dress appropriately and safely?
- Controlling body temperature – Does Doris feel cold? Is that why she is switching the gas fire on? If so, then what impact will switching off the gas have on Doris and what can be done to support her?
- Mobilising – How can nursing staff support Doris to move safely? This is closely linked, for Doris, with maintaining a safe environment; therefore similar questions around footwear, foot health, and handrails may need to be asked. There may also need to be a plan in place for if Doris does fall.
- Working and playing – Doris has always been busy and enjoys gardening; how can nursing staff support Doris to continue to be busy and to continue gardening in a safe way?
- Expressing sexuality – What support does Doris need to express her sexuality? What impact, if any, does this have on her care?
- Sleeping – Does Doris need any other support or aids at night to help her mobilise to the toilet or sleep safely in bed? What support does Doris need to get to bed?

- Dying – Does Doris have any specific wishes around end-of-life care should she become unwell? How may this affect her care now and in the future?

DO MODELS HAVE A VALUE IN MODERN NURSING?

Nursing care is delivered in a wide variety of settings, from acute intensive care to attending to a person in their own home. From the first contact with a new patient, to supporting long-term conditions and palliative and end-of-life care, Registered Nurses use processes and procedures to meet their patients' needs. Nursing undoubtedly changes over time, with research into different conditions and people's response to them, but also, we as Registered Nurses change over time, we evolve, we grow with experience, and this can also influence the way we adapt and work within nursing processes and how valuable nursing models are to our practice.

Registered Nurses must always deliver the fundamentals of care and each patient's dignity must be upheld along with their rights, wants, and needs. Registered Nurses are required to prioritise the people they serve at all times, providing compassionate person-centred care. The Nursing and Midwifery Council Code of Practice states that Registered Nurses must 'treat people with kindness, respect and compassion'.

NMC

THE CODE SAYS

1 **Treat people as individuals and uphold their dignity**
   To achieve this, you must:
   1.1 treat people with kindness, respect and compassion
   1.2 make sure you deliver the fundamentals of care effectively
   1.3 avoid making assumptions and recognise diversity and individual choice
   1.4 make sure that any treatment, assistance or care for which you are responsible is delivered without undue delay
   1.5 respect and uphold people's human rights

To achieve this in nursing practice, there must be processes, or nursing models, that can flex and stretch around the people Registered Nurses care for to provide a framework for care delivery.

However, it can be argued that some models encourage Registered Nurses to assess but don't specify what they should be assessing, and also that planning is vital but there is little guidance on how to write effective care plans. Nursing models are a theoretical construct and therefore do not provide specifics and because of this the Registered Nurse's understanding of the model and the application of it is key. Models are criticised by some in nursing as being of little value and celebrated by others as being vital to nursing practice.

In addition to this, it's worth noting that many modern nursing documentation booklets have multiple assessments which only require the Registered Nurse to add a tick or a cross to a box and there is limited opportunity to free text those areas where our patients don't neatly fit within the confines of the box unless using generic nursing notes. These documentation booklets seem to follow no nursing model and rely on Registered Nurses' own clinical judgement to either apply a model to their assessment, diagnosis, planning, implementation, and evaluation of care or not.

Registered Nurses must continuously consider their professional development within nursing and how their practice as a registrant can impact patient experience; therefore as a nursing student, you will be developing this skill, so ultimately, it's up to you to look at and reflect on your own practice and the value that nursing models may offer you.

What are your thoughts on nursing models and their value in your practice?

_____

_____

_____

_____

_____

_____

_____

LOOKING BEYOND NURSING-SPECIFIC MODELS

There are many other models used across healthcare and nursing that can have value to Registered Nurses, nursing and the people we care for.

TWEET

@ruth-rawson:

'The Health Belief model will inform my practice in primary care when trying to change behaviour. It guides you to identify and address threats (barriers) and raise awareness of the benefits of making a behaviour change. Very helpful! #WeNurses'

TWEET

@_jamilahhx:

'I do identify with Benner's Stages of Clinical Competence because as a Novice I do believe my ability to predict certain situations is limited due to my lack of experience in the field as I am a student. #WeNurses'

The PDSA (Plan, Do, Study, Act) Cycle is an example of a model that is not specifically aimed at nursing but is still relevant to nursing practice (Fig 6.2).

The need to change the delivery of healthcare to reduce cost and improve quality lends itself to the use of the PDSA cycle and this methodology is being used widely to drive forward quality improvement programs internationally in healthcare (Christoff 2018). PDSA cycles enable small but rapid changes to be made and this allows timely change, something that the NHS has been criticised for not achieving over the years. Small changes in clinical care delivery, for example, trialling a new ulcer dressing, are often easier to embed too, as they do not feel so overwhelming as, for example, big legislative or policy changes.

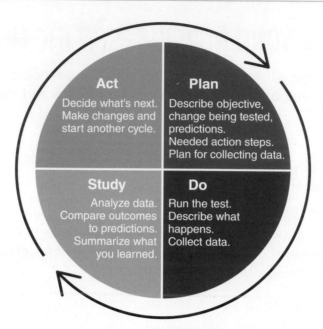

Figure 6.2   The PDSA cycle. (Eby, K (2021) The essential guide to PDSA: Models, worksheets and templates Smartsheet Available at https://www. smartsheet.com/content/plan-do-study-act-guide (last accessed 23/9/22).

Change is something all Registered Nurses not only have to learn to accept but also lead. It can be said that without change there can be no progress. Historically nursing was very task focused and in more recent times there has been a shift towards evidence-based, scientific nursing. Cutcliffe and Bassett (2003) found that within large health institutions changes at all levels can be made and shown to have real benefits to patient safety and quality care.

There are also tools, which are closely related to models, that are commonly used within nursing and support the delivery of care. The National Early Warning Scores (NEWS) are a great example of how a simple design can be easy to use and enhances Registered Nurses' ability to identify and respond to deteriorating patients (Fox and Elliott 2015). NHS England (2022) define NEWS as 'a tool developed by the Royal College of Physicians which improves the detection and response to clinical deterioration in adult patients and is a key element of patient safety and improving patient outcomes'.

Physiological parameter	Score						
	3	2	1	0	1	2	3
Respiration rate (per minute)	≤8		9–11	12–20		21–24	≥25
SpO₂ Scale 1 (%)	≤91	92–93	94–95	≥96			
SpO₂ Scale 2 (%)	≤83	84–85	86–87	88–92 ≥93 on air	93–94 on oxygen	95–96 on oxygen	≥94 on oxygen
Air or oxygen?		Oxygen		Air			
Systolic blood pressure (mmHg)	≤90	91–100	101–110	111–219			≥220
Pulse (per minute)	≤40		41–50	51–90	91–110	111–130	≥131
Conciousness				Alert			CVPU
Temperature (°C)	≤35.0		35.1–36.0	36.1–38.0	38.1–39.0	≥39.1	

Figure 6.3 INTEROPen (2019) National Early Warning Score (NEWS) 2 Available at https://nhsconnect.github.io/FHIR-NEWS2/index.html (last accessed 23/9/22).

The NEWS can easily be integrated within existing nursing documentation to enhance an existing model of care and improve the identification of early deterioration in patients (Fig 6.3).

What other models have you come across and how can you use them in your own practice?

_____

_____

_____

_____

_____

_____

The care environment and nursing models

Nursing is a diverse career, with many different areas of practice and specialties. If you asked a member of the public where Registered Nurses work, most of them would say 'in hospitals'; however, an increasing number of Registered Nurses work in community settings, primary care, and people's own homes. Even within hospital nursing there are many different specialist areas, and care delivered in the emergency department differs significantly from a rehabilitation ward, general medical, elective surgical, and so on. Then there are general practice nurses, district nurses, specialist community nurses, mental health and learning disability services both inpatient and community – the list goes on and on! It is important to consider how these diverse care environments can affect the use of nursing models and consider whether nursing models need to be adapted to meet the environmental needs of care delivery.

Think about all the different clinical care areas you know of/have worked in/had placements in – how are they different? How does this impact care?

_____

_____

_____

_____

_____

_____

_____

It's important for Registered Nurses to consider the environment in which they work. Florence Nightingale first identified the environment as being fundamental for health and healing – her premise was that clean air, clean water, light, and basic sanitation influenced the speed and success of recovery from illness. This thinking can be seen in theories today, for example, the theories underpinning infection prevention processes and aseptic techniques:

CASE STUDY

Healthcare-acquired infections can be very problematic to treat and recover from. Hart (2007) discussed the importance of the use of aseptic techniques to minimise the risk of healthcare-acquired infection for the patient while also protecting the Registered Nurse from being contaminated by a patient's bodily fluids. In addition to this the theory of aseptic techniques has evolved in line with research and development and the aseptic non-touch technique (ANTT) is currently being advocated as the most effective way to minimise healthcare-acquired infections (Rowley and Clare 2011), ensuring patients requiring dressings have the best health outcomes. The ANTT process can be easily integrated into existing nursing documentation and models.

Building on this, Nightingale also believed that nurses must use their brains, hearts, and hands to improve the environment and be sure to care for the patient's physical, emotional, and social needs – something which is still reflected in contemporary nursing practice as we strive to deliver holistic nursing care. For example:

The use of lighting and colour in dementia care has long been established as having beneficial effects for patients with dementia and some of the interventions for dementia care environments have actively demonstrated a decline in the use of sedative medication (Alzheimer's Society 2015). Ludden et al. (2019) found that the use of handrails to support people with dementia finding their way around units was beneficial and also reduced the risk of falls as there was something available to support people as they moved around the unit. When supporting people with dementia it is important to consider sensory processes and how to assess positive stimuli such as gardens, herbs, and pictures and be able to avoid negative stimuli such as strip lights and loud noises which may contribute to a negative experience for the person (Flemming, Kelly, and

Stillfried 2015). Flemming, Kelly, and Stillfried (2015) also acknowledged there was a range of preferences and responses from people with dementia and their carers in regard to what their priorities were for their environment. This ultimately improves the patient experience and reduces the risk of behavioural and psychological symptoms of dementia and this improves the nursing experience and job satisfaction.

In both examples, it is clear that the diverse nursing environments need to be considered when thinking about models and it's important for Registered Nurses to understand how models can be flexed and adapted to meet individual needs and wants. A nursing model can simply be a starting point from which to improve or deliver care and does not necessarily need to be taken and used word for word.

'We introduced a whole new care plan structure at Little Heath Care Home over a year ago, which helped us move to a far more holistic process. This has resulted in a change in the way we assess, plan, implement and evaluate care. The new care plan documentation followed elements of Roper, Logan and Tierney nursing model based on activities of daily living:

- *communication,*
- *breathing,*
- *eating and drinking,*
- *eliminating,*
- *personal cleansing and dressing,*
- *mobilising,*
- *expressing sexuality,*
- *sleeping*

The following elements were then added in:

- *pressure area/skin care*
- *specific worries and fears*

The dying element was omitted as it was felt when a person entered this phase of their life that another type of care plan was needed.

It was important that we were able to tie in work by Kitwoood around caring for people with dementia – considering his work on identity, life story, social psychology, neurological impairment, personality and life history.

- *emotional and psychological wellbeing plan*
- *nighttime wellbeing plan*
- *behavioural support plan*
- *life story*
- *how to support me*

This was a new way of working for staff at Little Heath as previously no model was used, and documents were placed randomly within care plans and not in clear themes. This new approach amalgamated two models which enables us to plan the most person-centred care possible for people living with dementia, taking into account all factors associated with their level of wellbeing.

The documentation we are using has allowed us to make significant changes and support people exhibiting distressed behaviours in order to identify the reasons why they may be behaving this way and to evaluate our interventions.

The new format is much less confusing for staff because it follows a clear process and easily indicates when further intervention is required and provides the opportunity for input from the whole care and nursing team.

We have been able to personalise the two models to our resident group giving us a comprehensive way to assess, plan, implement and evaluate care, especially for those living with a dementia'.

–Samantha Jenkins, Registered Nurse and Deputy Manager

There are an increasing number of Registered Nurses working in community settings and providing home-based care and with the development of Integrated Care Services (ICSs) across the health system this diversity will increase. Registered Nurses working in community-based roles play a vital role in health education, delivery of quality care, and making quality and safety improvements to care delivery (Hughes 2008). When providing care in a person's own home the Registered Nurse must be mindful that they need to explore adaptations to models of care to meet the individuals' holistic needs (Flemming 2015), and the balance needs to be found to ensure that health outcomes can be achieved and health maximised while considering the specific individual needs of the patient and respecting their autonomy and dignity. For example:

It is clear to see that Registered Nurses work in many environments which can influence the delivery of care and the choice of model to use or even adapt when providing care and nursing interventions.

Evidence-based nursing and models

Essential to the development of nursing practice is the use of evidence which influences how Registered Nurses and nursing students plan and deliver care. The success of evidence-based practice in nursing practice is dependent on the successful transfer of knowledge (Scott et al. 2012) and for knowledge transfer to be successful it is vital to use a number of methods to share it. Research findings can be shared across nursing and healthcare in a variety of ways, and these must be considered when planning to make changes to current practice or introduce new ways of working, specifically adaptations to nursing models.

NMC 6 Always practise in line with the best available evidence

As nursing practice, evidence, and research continue to evolve, so does the legislation we use to underpin our practices and in turn this has influenced nursing models, documentation, and processes. Alongside nursing evolution, our patient demographic is evolving too, and nursing is now seeing a significant difference in patient presentation, which continues to change and challenge. In the last decade there has been an increase in patients who have additional vulnerabilities, for example, long-term conditions such as COPD, deteriorating conditions such as dementia, and multiple comorbidities which can make the nursing process more complex. This makes nursing practice an ever-changing landscape and within this there are demands for excellence and meeting the needs of an increasingly complex patient group. A good example of this is around people with dementia and how they mobilise: in 2009 the Alzheimer's Association identified that people with dementia often engage in walking with purpose and Registered Nurses may try to stop this from happening because of falls risks, when supporting patients' movement may in fact be more beneficial for the patient. This is supported by the Alzheimer's Society (2015) which advocates personalised care plans, increased levels of observation, and best interest meetings with relatives. The question is, do contemporary nursing models allow this to happen? Or are they so focused on risk management that we focus on maintaining safety and avoiding falls as a priority and not consider so much what is psychologically better for the patient? This is where the application of a nursing model can help Registered Nurses to assess which is the most appropriate option for the patient, and in collaboration with the patient (or relatives when the patient lacks the capacity to consent themselves) this can result in a bespoke care plan which best meets the patient's needs.

Following a model can really support the development of nursing practice and remind Registered Nurses what information they need to be gaining from their patients in order to make that robust assessment and care plan. It helps Registered Nurses to consider the different elements within care delivery and identify and prioritise them. What is important for one patient will be different for another patient, and alongside that there are clinical priorities to consider too.

Models for nursing practice have been around for decades, as has the activities of daily living model mentioned earlier in this chapter and it can be argued that the Roper Logan Tierney model is still able to deliver in contemporary nursing as the fundamental principles on which it is based have not changed.

Another aspect to consider when exploring evidence-based nursing and nursing models is social determinants of health, which are important because they have been identified as influencing treatment options and recovery times. Social determinants of health are things like poverty, poor housing, unemployment, and social disconnectedness (Atkinson et al. 2013). Each of these social determinants requires consideration and application to a nursing model to maximise patient outcomes, and Registered Nurses have to seriously consider how factors external to care delivery impact care and treatment. For example:

CASE STUDY

A person living in poverty with diabetes may appear to be non-compliant with treatment in relation to dietary regime; however, the reality for that person is they are not able to afford the correct foodstuffs as advised by the Registered Nurse treating them. In this situation the nursing care depends on careful consideration of budget and what is realistic to expect of the patient. While there is limited evidence to support that the social determinants of health specifically impact health outcomes, they are part of a complex set of variables including genetic characteristics and lifestyle choices (Sheehan and Sheehan 2015).

Carey and Crammond (2015) have identified that when addressing issues relating to social determinants of health it is change in government policy which is seen as more powerful and effective than changes made at the service delivery level. However, it can also be argued that national policy change, for example, the implementation of the National Service Framework for Diabetes (Department of Health 2001), drives change at the point of service delivery. The introduction of the National Service Framework for Diabetes identified that every patient with a diagnosis of diabetes should have access to a diabetes clinic; this created specific diabetes nurse specialists who deliver on clinics across the UK.

> *'Standard 4: Clinical care of adults with diabetes 4. All adults with diabetes will receive high-quality care throughout their lifetime, including support to optimise the control of their blood glucose, blood pressure and other risk factors for developing the complications of diabetes'.*

> *(Department of Health 2001)*

The aim of the National Service Frameworks was to improve quality, minimise variation, and reduce health inequalities within the UK population. A key component of this was to ensure partnership working with the clinical team, including specialist nurses, and the patient. The development of nurse-led specialist clinics like the diabetic clinic requires

Registered Nurses to redesign existing models to tailor them to their patient population, ensuring the key diabetic standards are met while maintaining a holistic approach to assessment and ongoing care.

CASE STUDY

John is 54 and divorced. He lives alone in a 6th-floor flat with his dog and has type 1 diabetes which he was diagnosed with as a teenager. John has two adult children from his marriage but they live and work in different cities now and he does not have regular contact with them. John has not always complied with his diabetic regime and does not always attend appointments at the diabetic clinic. He frequently alters how much insulin he administers depending on what he is eating and does not always check his blood sugars. He has had 11 emergency department visits in the last 18 months due to poor regulation of his diabetes, including two admissions where he has been found in the street unresponsive. John admits to the triage nurse at his last emergency admission that since losing his job he has started drinking and is struggling to manage his finances. John was admitted to a medical ward for further assessment and stabilisation of his diabetes. On the ward John demonstrates that he has a good understanding of his condition and how to administer insulin and check his blood sugars. He also chooses a diabetic menu at mealtimes.

Nursing models and technology

In all healthcare provider settings, there are a myriad of nursing platforms and computerised systems to navigate – Lorenzo, Emis, Ormis, Portal, CRSS, Datix, Badgernet, synergie, Epex, Carefirst – to name but a few. Many of these platforms have the functionality to add assessments, documentation, and observations and digitalise patient care, in line with one of the core priorities for the NHS, which is to digitise care and connect technology to deliver a modern, seamless service for all patients (Hakim 2022). This dovetails with NHS England's Five Year Forward view which seeks to establish integrated care services which will deliver person-centred individualised care. The Care Quality Commission (2022) identifies that the main function of NHS services is the management of long-term conditions, and the new models of integrated care will support the effective delivery of these services.

There is, however, no template for what an integrated care plan should look like and which, if any, nursing model it should follow.

NHS England identify that a personalised care and support plan must meet the five criteria below:

1. People are central in developing and agreeing on their personalised care and support plan including deciding who is involved in the process.
2. People have proactive, personalised conversations which focus on what matters to them, paying attention to their needs and wider health and wellbeing.
3. People agree on the health and wellbeing outcomes they want to achieve, in partnership with the relevant professionals.
4. Each person has a sharable, personalised care and support plan which records what matters to them, their outcomes, and how they will be achieved.
5. People are able to formally and informally review their personalised care and support plan. (NHS England 2022)

However, for digitised care to truly work, it could be argued that the information technology (IT) systems within most healthcare providers must be updated. NHS IT systems have often been described as not being 'fit for purpose' and it is well known that patient platforms are not integrated and do not 'talk' with each other (Hakim 2022). This can be problematic within a single organisation, let alone regionally or nationally and the lack of IT communication between platforms can create gaps in care history and service provision and can negatively impact patient care.

For effective sharing of patient information between platforms to achieve integrated care, consideration must be given to General Data Protection Regulation (GDPR) and how this information can be shared legally and with patient consent. This important legal consideration may account for some of the ongoing delays in developing healthcare IT systems which are fully integrated.

All of this means that nursing care during this digital transformation often sits under medical models or data-driven models of care and there is a reliance on Registered Nurses and nursing students to have a working knowledge of nursing models and apply them to their own individual practice.

CONCLUSION

The evolution of nursing has been and continues to be remarkable, and as such it remains an ever-changing landscape, adapting to meet the needs of the people Registered Nurses serve. What is acceptable practice changes as new research and evidence emerges to guide us as Registered Nurses in shaping our practice and how we achieve the health outcomes for our patients changes alongside this. New terminology and processes within nursing models are constantly being introduced and developed, and alongside this, new models, tools, and technology are being introduced into healthcare, all of which influence nursing models and the application of them in practice.

TWEET

@wlasinclair:

'I think it's important to learn about different nursing models and consider how they can be used to guide practice...but do we need more contemporary models or are they still relevant to our practice in 2021?'

In the increasingly complex world of nursing and healthcare nursing students need to begin to understand nursing models to help them care for and support patients across many settings.

Now you have finished this chapter. Please make notes on what you have learner.

_____

_____

_____

_____

_____

_____

_____

_____

_____

_____

_____

_____

_____

_____

_____

_____

_____

_____

_____

_____

REFERENCES

Aggleton, P. Chalmers, H. (1986) Nursing Models and the Nursing Process. Macmillan, London.

Alzheimer's Society (2009) Facts for the Media [online] Available at: https://www.alzheimers.org.uk/site/scripts/documents_info.php?documentID=535&pageNumber=2 (last accessed November 2021).

Alzheimer's Society (2015) Dementia Care Practice Recommendations for Assisted Living Residences and Nursing Homes [online] Available at: https://www.alz.org/national/documents/brochure_DCPRphases1n2.pdf (last accessed November 2021).

Ambrose, A.F., Geet, P., Hausdorff, J.M. (2013) Risk factors for falls among older adults: A review of the literature. Maturitas 75(1) pp. 51–61.

Atkinson, D., Boulter, P., Hebron, C., Moulster, G. (2013) The Health Equalities Framework – An Outcomes Framework Based in the Determinants of Health Inequalities. National Development Team of Inclusion.

Barrett, D., Wilson, B., Woollands, A. (2012) Care Planning: A Guide for Nurses. 2nd Edition. Routledge, London.

Care Quality Commission (2022) New Care Models [online] Available at: https://www.cqc.org.uk/what-we-do/coordinated-care/new-care-models (last accessed August 2022).

Carey, G., Crammond, B. (2015) Systems change for the social determinants of health. British Medical Council Public Health 15 p. 662.

Casey A. (1988) A partnership with child and family. Senior Nurse 8(4) p. 8.

Catalano J.T. (1996) Contemporary Professional Nursing. Davis, Philadelphia.

Christoff, P. (2018) Running PDSA cycles. Current Problems in Pediatric and Adolescent Health Care 48(8) pp. 198–201.

Cutcliffe, J.R., Bassett, C. (2003) Introducing change in nursing: The case of research. Journal of Nursing Management 5(4) pp. 241–247.

Department of Health (2001) National Service Framework: Diabetes Crown London.

Eby, K. (2021) The essential guide to PDSA: Models, worksheets and templates *Smartsheet* Available at https://www.smartsheet.com/content/plan-do-study-act-guide (last accessed September 2022).

Edemekong, P.F., Bomgaars, D.L., Sukumaran, S., Levy, S.B. (2017) Activities of Daily Living [online] Available at: Activities of Daily Living - Abstract - Europe PMC (last accessed March 2022).

Flemming, R., Kelly, F., Stillfried, G. (2015) 'I want to feel at home': Establishing what aspects of environmental design are important to people with dementia nearing the end of life. BMC Palliative Care 14(26).

Fox, A. Elliott, N. (2015) Early Warning Scores: A sign of deterioration in patients and systems. Nursing Management 22(1) pp. 26–31.

Friedman, A. (2012) Continuing Professional Development – Lifelong Learning of Millions. Routledge, London.

General Data Protection Regulation (2016) [online] Available at: https://gdpr-info.eu/ (last accessed August 2022).

Hakim, R. (2022) The Digital Health and Care Plan: What Must It Address? NHS Confederation [online] Available at https://www.nhsconfed.org/publications/digital-health-and-care-plan (last accessed August 2022).

Hart, S. (2007) Using an aseptic technique to reduce the risk of infection. Nursing Standard 21(47) pp. 43–48.

Holland, K., Jenkins, J. (2019) Applying the Roper-Logan-Tierney Model in Practice. 3rd Edition. Elsevier, London.

Hughes, R. (2008) Patient Safety and Quality: An Evidence-Based Handbook for Nurses. Volume 1. Agency for Healthcare Research and Quality, USA.

INTEROPen (2019) National Early Warning Score (NEWS) 2 Available at: https://nhsconnect. github.io/FHIR-NEWS2/index.html (last accessed September 2022).

Ludden, G.D.S., van Rompay, T.J.L., Niedderer, K., Tournier, I. (2019) Environmental design for dementia care – Towards more meaningful experiences through design. Maturitas 128 pp. 10–16.

McKenna, H., Pajinkihar, M., Murphy, F. (2014) Fundamentals of Nursing Models, Theories and Practice. Wiley, London.

Moulster, G., Griffiths T. (2012) Implementation of a new framework for practice. Learning Disability Practice 15(7) pp. 21–26.

Murphy, F., Williams, A., Pridmore, J.A. (2010) Nursing models and contemporary nursing 1: Their development, uses and limitations. Nursing Times 106(23) [online] Available at: https://www.nursingtimes.net/roles/nurse-educators/nursing-models-and-contemporary-nursing-1-their-development-uses-and-limitations-15-06-2010/ (last accessed February 2022).

NHS England (2022a) National Early Warning Score (NEWS) Available at: https://www.england.nhs.uk/ourwork/clinical-policy/sepsis/nationalearlywarningscore/ (last accessed September 2022).

NHS England (2022b) Personalised Care and Support Planning [online] Available at: https://www.england.nhs.uk/ourwork/patient-participation/patient-centred/planning/ (last accessed August 2022).

NHS England (2019) Five Year Forward View [online] Available at: https://www.england.nhs.uk/five-year-forward-view/ (last accessed August 2022).

Orem, D. (1991) Dorothea Orem's Self-Care Theory [online] Available at: http://currentnursing.com/nursing_theory/self_care_deficit_theory.html (last accessed September 2015).

Pearson, A. Vaughan, B. Fitzgerald, M. (2005) Nursing Models for Practice. 3rd Edition. Butterworth Heinemann, London.

Perry, A., Potter, P., Ostendorf, W. (2014) Clinical Nursing Skills and Techniques. 8th Edition. Elsevier.

Peplau, H. (2015) Hildegard Peplau – Nursing Theory [online] Available at: http://nursing-theory.org/nursing-theorists/Hildegard-Peplau.php (last accessed September 2022).

Roper, N., Logan, W., Tierney, A. (2000) The Roper-Logan-Tierney Model of Nursing. Churchill Livingstone, London.

Rowley, S., Clare, S. (2011) ANTT: A standard approach to aseptic technique. Nursing Times 107(36) pp. 12–14.

Sheehan, P., Sheehan, M. (2015) Caring about the social determinants of health. America Journal of Bioethics. 15(3) pp. 48–50.

Toney-Butler, J. Thayer, J. (2022) Nursing Process. National Library of Medicine [online] Available at: https://www.ncbi.nlm.nih.gov/books/NBK499937/#:,:text=These%20are%20 assessment%2C%20diagnosis%2C%20planning%2C%20implementation%2C%20 and%20evaluation.&text=Assessment%20is%20the%20first%20step,data% 20collection%3B%20subjective%20and%20objective (last accessed August 2022).

Torrens, C., Campbell, P., Hoskins, G., Strachan, H., Wells, M., Cunningham, M., Bottone, H., Polson, R., Maxwell, M. (2020) Barriers and facilitators to the implementation of the advanced nurse practitioner role in primary care settings: A scoping review. International Journal of Nursing Studies 104(2020) 103443.

Wayne, G. (2022) The Nursing Process: A comprehensive Guide. *NurseLabs* Available at: https://nurseslabs.com/nursing-process/ (last accessed September 2022).

TWITTER REFERENCES

@_jamilahhx [Twitter] Available at: https://twitter.com/_jamilahhx/status/13693848669 58221314?s=20&t=p-Pfm05nDO7JIAHfTrYoqQ (last accessed September 2022).

@KirstyEverett3 (2021) [Twitter] Available at: https://twitter.com/KirstyEverett3/status/ 1369392654576934924?s=20&t=SS07zCBgl_ystBfXZmK3dQ (last accessed September 2022).

@KirstyEverett3 (2021) [Twitter] Available at: https://twitter.com/KirstyEverett3/status/ 1369387990854889475?s=20&t=I4CdIAWf1sqCcOzb62OwDw (last accessed September 2022).

@ruth_rawson (2021) [Twitter] Available at: https://twitter.com/ruth_rawson/status/ 1369385386766647296?s=20&t=x1tGQtG2Y-XZDD0∠4OMfSA (last accessed September 2022).

@wenurses (2021) [Twitter] Available at: https://twitter.com/WeNurses/status/1369386 284855267342?s=20&t=I4CdIAWf1sqCcOzb62OwDw (last accessed September 2022).

@wlasinclair (2021) [Twitter] Available at: https://twitter.com/wlasinclair/status/1369390 354701692933?s=20&t=SS07zCBgl_ystBfXZmK3dQ (last accessed September 2022).

@wlasinclair (2021) [Twitter] Available at: https://twitter.com/wlasinclair/status/1369392 233972178954?s=20&t=vsWgN-XlsPtxw5VIrc5YSw (last accessed September 2022).

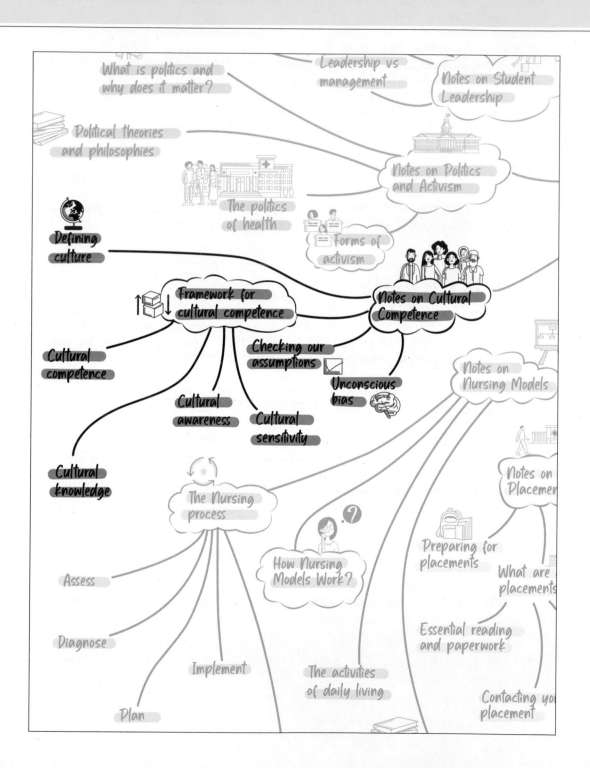

NOTES ON CULTURAL COMPETENCE

Eula Eudolah Miller (She/Her) ■ Rebecca Lowe (She/Her)
■ Gayatri Nambiar-Greenwood (She/Her)
■ Hetal Patel (He/Him)

INTRODUCTION

Developing cultural competence is a life-long, continuous process. The aim of this chapter is to provide insight into how the gap between theory and practice can be bridged, from the knowing to the doing. It shifts the understanding of cultural competence from theoretical frameworks to a process of self-awareness that encourages parity and equity within relationships, where the uniqueness in all individuals is celebrated.

Deeper understanding of this topic and reflect on how to grow into becoming a culturally competent nursing student. This process encourages the exploration of one's own biases, which may bring up feelings of discomfort. Such reflection will help enhance self-awareness and is part of the journey.

The infographic displayed in Figure 7.1, adapted from one of the many cultural competence frameworks, has informed the approach to structuring this chapter. It contains all the terms that a culturally competent nursing student has to consider when developing relationships with patients. To treat someone in a culturally competent manner is to avoid treating everyone in the same way or to base their delivery of care on the norms, practices, and beliefs of the majority culture.

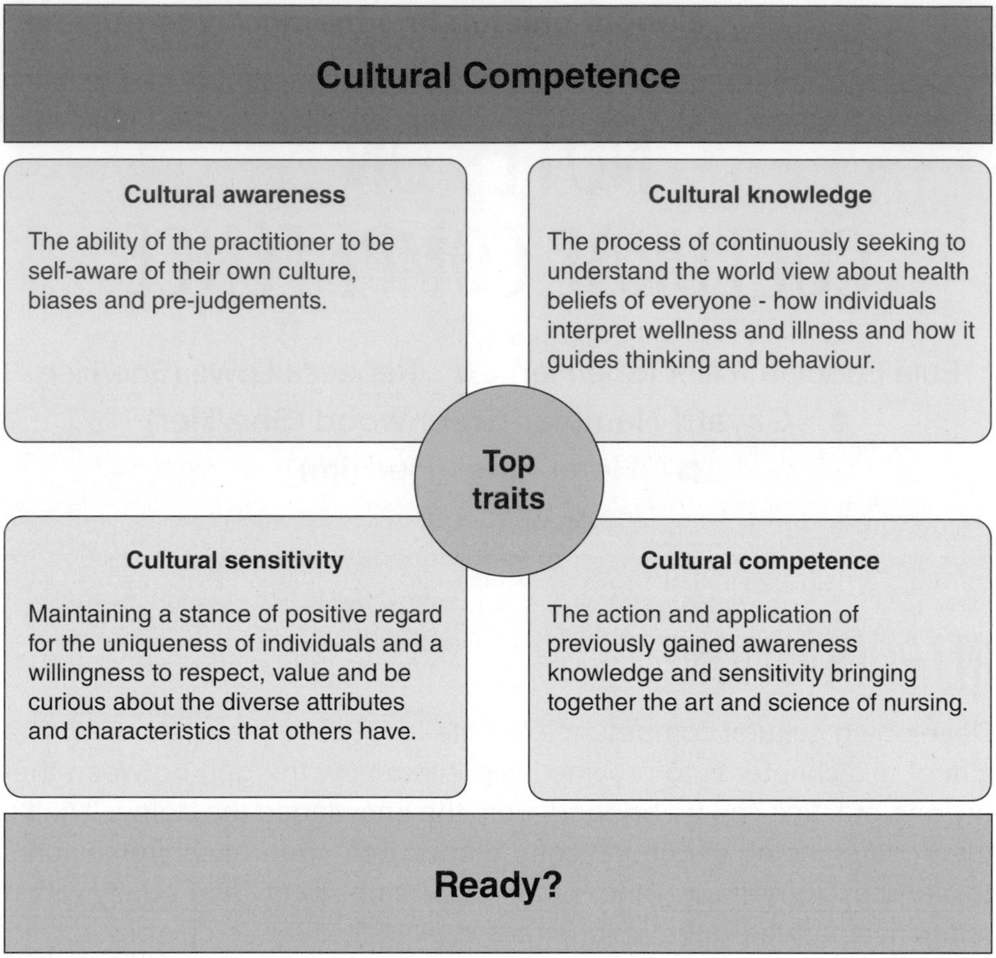

Cultural Competence

Cultural awareness

The ability of the practitioner to be self-aware of their own culture, biases and pre-judgements.

Cultural knowledge

The process of continuously seeking to understand the world view about health beliefs of everyone - how individuals interpret wellness and illness and how it guides thinking and behaviour.

Top traits

Cultural sensitivity

Maintaining a stance of positive regard for the uniqueness of individuals and a willingness to respect, value and be curious about the diverse attributes and characteristics that others have.

Cultural competence

The action and application of previously gained awareness knowledge and sensitivity bringing together the art and science of nursing.

Ready?

Figure 7.1   The Papadopoulos, Tilki and Taylor Model for Developing Cultural Competence.

NMC Behaviours/standards related to being a culturally competent nursing student

NMC

THE CODE SAYS

1: Treat people as individuals and uphold their dignity.

To achieve this, you must:

1.3 Avoid making assumptions and recognise diversity and individual choice

1.5 Respect and uphold people's human rights

1.14 Provide and promote non-discriminatory, person centred and sensitive care at all times, reflecting on people's values and beliefs, diverse backgrounds, cultural characteristics, language requirements, needs and preferences, taking account of any need for adjustments

Professional Standard 7: Communicate clearly.

To achieve this, you must:

7.3 Use a range of verbal and non-verbal communication methods, and consider cultural sensitivities, to better understand and respond to people's personal and health needs

Professional Standard 20: Uphold the reputation of your profession at all times.

To achieve this, you must:

20.3 Be aware at all times of how your behaviour can affect and influence the behaviour of other people

Culturally competent care is the ethical, legal, and moral stipulations for all levels of Registered Nurses and is mandated by the Nursing and Midwifery Council (NMC, 2018). Maps the related professional standards and behaviours that nursing students must uphold.

What does the word 'Culture' mean to you?

_____

_____

_____

_____

_____

_____

DEFINING CULTURE

A good place to start is by looking at a broad definition of culture. According to Cecil Helman (2007), culture is a set of adopted customs or traditions, which informs society how to view their own world and how to experience it emotionally. For example, an obvious custom in the UK is the tendency to naturally form queues in shops, or to use the custom of drinking tea to signify sharing or giving comfort.

Such customs of culture also inform those connections to symbols, language, art, and literature that are passed on to the next generation. This sustains past rituals and shared identities. For example, there is a tendency to share customs and rituals that parents practised at home, from the way holidays are celebrated to the ceremonies used in grieving. Culture is not just about festivals, food, and dress that people who are different (such as by ethnicity, nationality, religion, amongst others) have. The premise from which this chapter is written is that there is a need to recognise that everyone is a cultural being and is affected by the world around them, even when the person is part of the majority population and thinks that their culture is normal.

How would you define yourself culturally? Do you find it difficult to describe yourself culturally? Do you often say: 'I don't have any culture'? We can all find it hard to describe ourselves culturally if we are part of the majority population in a village/town/city/country. Try looking at culture in a broader way. Think of the football team you support. The things that you and your friends do all the time together, say, getting ready on a Friday night to go out or even the way we celebrate New Year's Eve, irrespective of our background.

Make some notes on how you would define yourself culturally

_____

_____

_____

_____

_____

_____

A FRAMEWORK OF CULTURAL COMPETENCE

There are numerous definitions of cultural competence but the one chosen to work with is the seminal definition by Papadopoulos, Tilki, and Taylor (2006:10) Figure 7.2. They say that cultural competence is '*A process and an output, which results from the synthesis of knowledge and skills that we acquire during our personal and professional lives and to which we are constantly adding*'. The significance of this definition is that it sees that the skills required to become culturally competent are based more on the co-produced relationship between yourself and the patient. It questions the approach where the nursing student is seen as the expert professional, and the other person is 'only' the patient.

Cultural competence is not an end product that a nursing student or any health and social care professional is presented with at the end of their training. Rather, it is an ongoing dynamic process of person-centredness. Papadopoulos' (2018) definition considers cultural competence as the

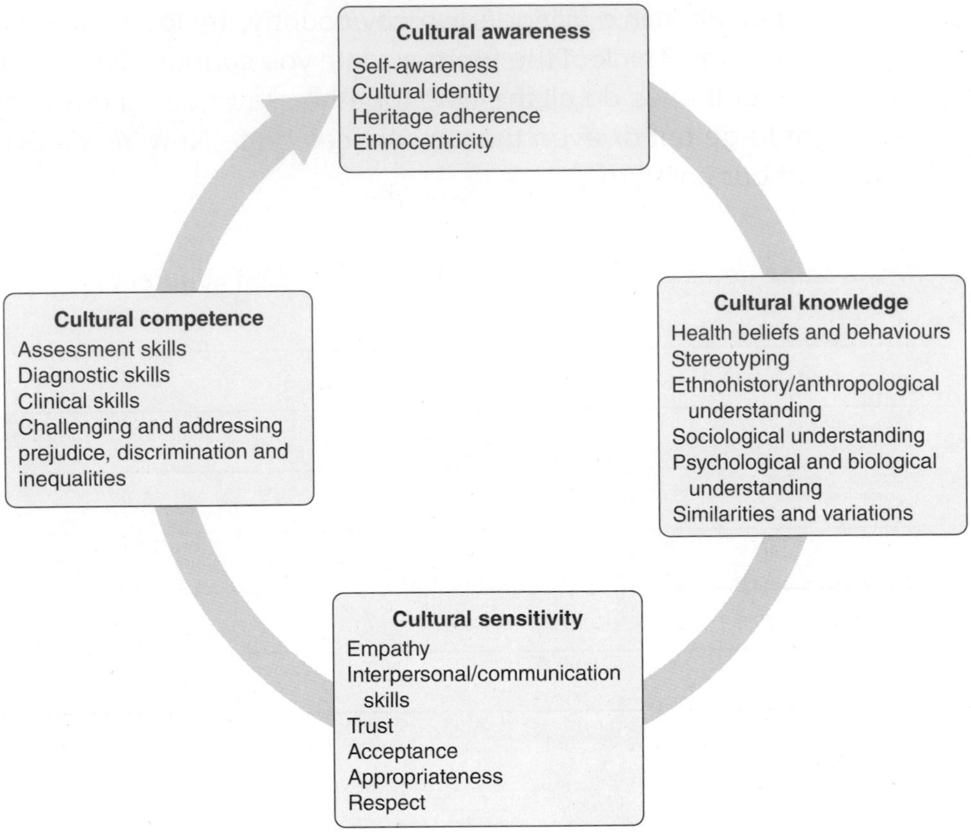

Cultural awareness
Self-awareness
Cultural identity
Heritage adherence
Ethnocentricity

Cultural knowledge
Health beliefs and behaviours
Stereotyping
Ethnohistory/anthropological
  understanding
Sociological understanding
Psychological and biological
  understanding
Similarities and variations

Cultural sensitivity
Empathy
Interpersonal/communication
  skills
Trust
Acceptance
Appropriateness
Respect

Cultural competence
Assessment skills
Diagnostic skills
Clinical skills
Challenging and addressing
prejudice, discrimination and
inequalities

Figure 7.2   A Framework of Cultural Competence (Papadopoulos, Tilki and Taylor, 2006).

capacity to deliver holistic health and social care by considering people's cultural beliefs, behaviours, and needs. This framework structures cultural competence as an ongoing process which, as outlined in the flow chart below, includes: cultural awareness, cultural knowledge, cultural sensitivity, and final cultural competence.

The process is about BECOMING culturally competent rather than BEING culturally competent. It's a learning journey. It's about being holistic in the way an individual is seen. Try to be interested and curious about the uniqueness of the patient being looked after, even if they look or share an ethnicity with you. Don't assume. Get to know the person or individual while suspending the stereotypes (e.g. colour, age, gender, ethnicity etc.). This requires the nursing student to be in the 'here and now' situation, with that person. This affords the patient full focus and attention, facilitating active listening necessary for a comprehensive holistic assessment to be undertaken.

Now that a definition and framework for cultural competence has been considered, let's work through the different elements of becoming a culturally competent nursing student, starting with 'Cultural Awareness'.

Cultural awareness

It would be very difficult to be a culturally competent nursing student without being self-aware. Self-awareness also includes being conscious of ethnocentrisms (comparing other cultures according to the preconceptions and standards of one's own culture). This begins with thinking about personal value base and beliefs. This is because the way cultural identity is constructed and internalised consequently influences what is thought of, and behaviour towards each patient's health beliefs and practices. Being self-aware of those factors and the conscious lens by which we see the patient is an effective platform in the process of cultural awareness. This also reduces stereotyping and promotes person-centredness. Being self-aware is not an absence of mistakes but the ability to learn, think, review, and refine them.

So, what can you do if you meet a person who seems to be very different from you? Ask yourself:

- Have I already made assumptions about this person?
- Where did those assumptions come from?
- Is it fair for me to hold an assumption of this person, based on my conventions from a previous situation or patient?
- Is it something I have heard or seen, that is: what the media says about the group this person represents?
- Did I speak to them in a way that was either rude, derogatory, or patronising?
- Did I attribute their mistake/lack of knowing to a personal characteristic unique to them (such as religion, ethnicity, disability), rather than a lack of their understanding of the situation?
- Am I avoiding this patient because they don't speak English well/are not verbal/ask too many questions?
- Have I attempted to speak to them in ways that do not just use verbal skills?

- Am I not happy about being asked all these questions because I feel I should know everything, or I want patients just to accept the care they are receiving?
- What does holding onto these assumptions do for me, in my relationship with this patient?

'As a first-year nursing student working on a respiratory ward, I was asked to check on a patient in one of the side rooms. On entering the patient's room, I introduced myself and then started to make conversation to start to build an initial relationship. After asking their name and how they were feeling that morning, I asked where they were from. The patient asked immediately in a frustrated manner "Why are you asking me that?" Inwardly, I was mortified that I had inadvertently offended the patient. I responded immediately by apologising for causing any offence and that I was asking purely out of interest. The patient challenged me and said, "do I ask that of everyone?" They went on to say that they get asked that question a lot and they wonder if it's because of the colour of their skin. We ended up having an honest, open and constructive conversation and I am forever grateful to this patient for bringing this to my attention. I reflected afterwards whether I do "unconsciously" ask more patients who are "different" to me about their background/origins. I have always been interested in learning about people's stories/journeys and it's part of the reason I'm studying to be a Registered Nurse. So, while I know my intentions are good, I want to become more self-aware of my own unconscious biases and to become more culturally aware/competent so that I can be more empathetic and to aim for being completely non-discriminatory in my practice – treating everyone as an individual. I know this is a continuous learning journey. I aim to come from a place of compassionate understanding and to quote Brené Brown "I'm here to get it right, not be right"!'

– Rebecca Lowe, nursing student

How individuals see themselves and those different from them is dependent on each person's personal experiences and views, which have the ability to influence our cultural conditioning. Life learning and experience frame the understanding of people who appear different.

Therefore, it is possible that a number of nursing students listening to one conversation or watching the same event will see, hear, and interpret different things. Each person's perception remains selective as there is a tendency to project one's own qualities onto others.

Checking Our Assumptions

If you were watching this from afar: what might they be saying to each other? What is the main emotion from either person? What makes you think that? Ask someone else to take a look at this picture and ask them what they see.

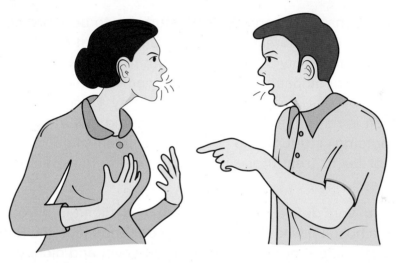

Write your thoughts here

_____

_____

_____

_____

_____

_____

_____

Viewing the picture above, how long did it take you to answer the questions? What informed your decisions? Did the person you asked see the same things as you? Is there an alternative story to the one you first had?

It is important not to make assumptions in day-to-day practice. While it is not possible to know everything about the many types of cultures present within our society today, it is possible to be aware of the varying cultural beliefs/values that could influence an individual's behaviour and to help question assumptions or pre-judgements about others.

Raising awareness amongst nursing students to be more conscious of the need to be culturally competent is important for all because it strengthens the ability to deliver care that is equitable, respectful, and dignified for all patients. As professionals, it ensures the uniqueness of the patient along their health journey. Despite unconscious bias, which is natural to human nature, having cultural competence allows nursing students to put those unchecked assumptions aside in order to treat those who require help in a person-centred manner.

How would you define equity, respect, and dignity? If you were a patient in a hospital who was completely dependant on the Registered Nurses how could they show you equity, respect and dignity.

In the following section there is a case study for you to read and consider the questions set at the end of each case study.

CASE STUDY

Abigail is a Registered Nurse who has just admitted Mrs Patel to her Assessment Unit for overnight observations due to Mrs Patel experiencing chest pains. She is currently being examined by Dr Jones; however, Mrs Patel is only able to communicate using some English and is therefore unable to explain clearly where her pain is just saying it is all over her chest. Abigail realises that Mrs Patel speaks very little English and thus is a poor history provider. She notices that she is not really being listened to by Dr Jones. He suggests that she has indigestion. Abigail urgently organises for the on-call interpreter and orders Mrs Patel an ECG. She does this because she has heard that non-native English-speaking patients may not be able to describe pain in the same way as those for whom this is their first language. Consequently, some conditions can go untreated and is the cause for increased morbidity in these groups.

The ECG shows that Mrs Patel has had a myocardial infarction and requires urgent treatment. With the help of an interpreter, the doctor is then able to ask, prescribe, and plan her treatment.

Consider:

Imagine you are in the Accident and Emergency department, in a foreign country, where you do not speak the language.

1. How would you know if the Registered Nurse in charge of your care empathises with you?
2. What type of verbal and non-verbal skills would she/he display that would reduce your anxiety?
3. What tools/assistance could the Registered Nurse put in place to ensure that safe care is delivered?
4. Think back to a time when you cared for a person who either did not share a language with you or was non-verbal (e.g. sign language user). How could you have improved the way you communicated with them?

_____

_____

_____

_____

_____

_____

Some things you may wish to consider:

Here the focus is on interpersonal and non-verbal skills. Registered Nurses, sometimes, when they can't communicate verbally or are faced with a sensitive issue, may avoid the patient. Being present and focused on the patient will show empathy. Actions such as a genuine smile, eye contact, a soft tone of voice (even when they don't understand), and your presence, despite lack of comprehension, are important.

- Contacting an interpreter should take precedence, or someone who may speak the same language. Although avoiding asking families to interpret is normal practice, they can be used for ensuring you have enough information to keep them safe (medication, general history etc., and taking down a few words that will help you communicate and provide basic care)

Exploring Unconscious Bias

Unconscious bias refers to those automatic pre-judgements that are made without thinking, such as stereotypes, racism, or sexism. Assumptions are made as soon as we set eyes on someone and are unavoidable, even there is no intention of being discriminatory. Examples of these can include 'all overweight people are lazy or greedy', 'Black men are aggressive', and 'all British are reserved and have a stiff upper lip'. Such unconscious biases can lead to careless ways of discriminating against others and is often unrealised by those who perpetuate it.

Think of a time when someone made a biased assumption about you. Also, think of a time when you made a judgement about someone and were proved wrong.

Unchecked unconscious biases do not only impact at an individual level, but they also have ramifications on wider health outcomes for all communities. Such examples from the UK include:

- White male physicians not effectively treating Black people with sickle cell anaemia in crisis due to the assumption of drug abuse amongst Black people (Beach et al., 2021)
- Assumptions made by health professionals that individuals who receive benefits and single parents are less intelligent and less likely to comply with health advice (Volmert et al., 2016)
- Men from traveller families assumed to be alcoholics (Francis, 2009)
- Assumptions that self-harmers are attention-seeking (Lloyd, 2018)
- Women presenting with cardiac heart disease symptoms pointedly being less likely than men to receive diagnosis, referral, and treatment, due to misdiagnosis of stress/anxiety (Garcia et al., 2017)
- Assumptions that individuals with a mental health diagnosis are not able to make rationale or competent decisions (Clarke et al., 2018)

Unconscious bias can manifest in a number of ways. The table below considers some of the different bias categories we all have but need to be aware of in order to be an effective nursing student.

Recognition of unconscious bias can leave us feeling uncomfortable as practitioners. So, what can we learn from this feeling of discomfort? We could:

A. Ignore it
B. Become defensive or hostile about it, and blame others
C. Rationalise and condone the biases
D. Acknowledge and reflect on it, in order to move forward as a culturally competent practitioner

DIFFERENT CATEGORIES OF BIAS

Ethnocentricity	To view one's own group, abilities, ethnicity, or nationality as comparatively superior to others	She wears a hijab, so she can't have as much freedom as I do/there's no point in explaining the condition to that patient; he is not very well educated or smart enough to understand
Cultural other	This comes from an imagined idea of difference, either superior or inferior to the cultural self-identity that may represent the normal	Fat people do not need stylish clothes; they just need to lose weight
Intercultural Communication Apprehension	A fear or anxiety associated with either real or anticipated communication with people from different groups, especially cultural and/or ethnic groups, which becomes ingrained with persistent negative views from media, society, or politics. This can result in an overly policed and inappropriate political correctness	That Asian lady doesn't speak English, so I will order her a Halal meal because I don't want to offend her
Unconscious bias/ implicit bias	Unsupported judgements or prejudice against a person or a group that, if unchecked, can have an impact on health and social care in matters of equity, diversity, and inclusion: forms of unconscious bias:	See examples below

DIFFERENT CATEGORIES OF BIAS—cont'd

Affinity bias refers to when you unconsciously and only prefer people who share qualities with you or someone you like. It occurs because your brain sees them as familiar and relatable, and we all want to be around people we can relate to; however, this can exclude others or stop you from hearing another perspective

I prefer nurses who are trained in the UK only because we are trained to very high standards and patients can understand them speaking English

Confirmation bias
We tend to remember and pay more attention to information that confirms our pre-existing beliefs. Also we can give more weight to information that is presented to us earlier rather than later despite evidence otherwise

All patients with dementia are confused, aggressive, and difficult to care for

Conformity bias
Conformity bias happens when your views are swayed too much by those of other people. It occurs because we all seek acceptance from others — we want to hold opinions and views that our community accepts

I better not say anything even if that nurse is being racist, because I have to work here with her every day/I want her to like me/I am choosing to pick my battles

Attribution bias refers to how you perceive your actions and those of others. Fundamental attribution error is the belief that, while our own actions can be explained by circumstances, others' behaviours are explained by their traits and personalities

I lost my temper with my nursing student because I had a really hard day/he lost his temper with the nursing student because he's a bully

Continued

DIFFERENT CATEGORIES OF BIAS—cont'd

Beauty bias
We all unconsciously notice people's appearances and associate them with their personality. Appearances are deemed important, particularly in a workplace setting, as they reflect on professionalism and self-awareness.
Many of us judge others too harshly based on their physical attractiveness or are unable to see beauty in the ways we have conformed to accepting what is considered beautiful

Oh my goodness, have you seen all her tattoos and her pink hair? She cannot possibly be a professional nurse

Cultural knowledge

The second stage, cultural knowledge, can be achieved in a number of ways. For example, even when patients seem to be like the person caring for them, assumptions or stereotypes of the needs and wants should not be made. Meaningful contact with people from different walks of life can enhance knowledge around their health beliefs and behaviours. A personal appreciation of the emotions around Intercultural Communication Apprehension (the fear or anxiety associated with interaction with people from different groups, especially different cultural or ethnic groups) can enhance open and honest discussion. A culturally competent nursing student will also be aware of the influence of professional power and make links between personal position and structural inequalities. For example, the uniform worn can cause patients to automatically assume that nursing students have all the knowledge pertaining to health matters. However, if a patient has lived with a condition for years, they may actually be the expert at what improves or worsens their condition.

It is important as a nursing student, in addition to building cultural awareness, to also build one's own knowledge/understanding of different cultures to be able to implement and tailor the care that is given.

 TIP

The following resources are a good starting point:

RCN (2019) guidance on expressing religious beliefs
RCN (2011) guidance on Spirituality in Nursing Care

 'When I was working on the ward, we were doing the usual morning routine and I was responsible for handing out breakfast to the patients in my bay. When collecting the plates an hour later, I noticed that Eunice [not the patient's real name], a bedbound 82 year old lady of West Indian origin hadn't touched her breakfast. I asked her why she didn't want her breakfast and she said that she and others from her West Indian community don't eat anything before brushing their teeth.

This gave me food for thought in terms of how I, as a nursing student caring for Eunice, can adapt the often-inflexible routines on the ward so they are more person-centred and culturally sensitive of the needs of others'.

– Gaynor Barber, nursing student

Cultural sensitivity

The third stage, cultural sensitivity, is how nursing students view those in their care. Weissman et al. (2017) express that unless clients are considered partners, culturally sensitive care cannot be achieved. This includes positive regard toward patients that have limited health literacy or some form of disability. To have positive regard is to have an attitude of caring, acceptance, and valuing the other person irrespective of their behaviour and without regard to differences or otherness. The expectation of patients as passive recipients is more likely to indicate that nursing students are using their power in an oppressive way.

Equal partnerships involve trust, acceptance, and respect, as well as facilitation and negotiation. It encourages the building of relationships, reciprocity, hearing, and sharing views as important as the physical care we give.

The figure 7.3 below shows an example of the principles of co-production.

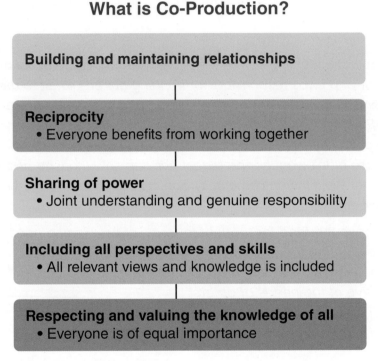

What is Co-Production?

Building and maintaining relationships

Reciprocity
• Everyone benefits from working together

Sharing of power
• Joint understanding and genuine responsibility

Including all perspectives and skills
• All relevant views and knowledge is included

Respecting and valuing the knowledge of all
• Everyone is of equal importance

Figure 7.3   Principles of Co-Production. (Image from Walker, 2019.)

Cultural competence

Cultural competence is the fourth stage. This is the action and application of previously gained awareness, knowledge, and sensitivity. It brings together the art and science of nursing. Attention is given to adjusting practical skills such as assessment of need, clinical diagnosis, and other caring skills to the patient. It is critical that the nursing student recognises and openly challenges all forms of discrimination and oppressive practice that can hinder a patient from getting equitable care. It is important to remember that when caring, understanding and engaging in a competent way for patients with similar characteristics, it is also key to be mindful of their unique differences too.

As discussed at the beginning of the chapter, there are some other concepts that are worth knowing about when starting the journey to becoming a culturally competent nursing student. These concepts are:

- **Cultural desire**: The motivation of nursing students to want to care for their diverse population with equal enthusiasm and creativity. It differentiates the 'want to care' from 'need to care' and focuses on the attribute of respectful, non-patronising curiosity.
- **Cultural skill**: The ability to collect relevant cultural information when patients attend with health complaints from a range of sources (the patient, guidebooks, internet), all while maintaining the individuality of the person. It focuses on the ability to undertake health assessments with an appreciation of the physical, biological, spiritual, and psychological variations between different groups. This should be done with the knowledge that we are naturally biased and can easily make assumptions.
- **Cultural encounters**: The process of the nursing student positively engaging with patients from *all* culturally diverse backgrounds but at the same time appreciating that cultural diversity includes patients from the majority or minority populations or those who look just like you. It is important to note that even if the patient comes from the same background as you (same religion, ethnicity, sexuality, town, country), they will have differences and unique requirements and you must be careful not to make assumptions.

CASE STUDY

Sue is a 65-year-old farmer who whilst recovering from cancer treatment at home has developed a cellulitis of her leg. She has been admitted to your ward and is on enforced bed rest. Mrs Malik, the patient across the room from her, is also on bedrest. Mrs Malik's daughters are allowed outside visiting hours but when Sue asks if she can have her visitors outside visiting hours, she is told that she has no cultural reason for it.

Consider:

1. Why do you think the staff felt that Sue's need for having visitors was less important than Mrs Malik's?
2. In denying Sue some comfort in a personally challenging time, what are Sue's cultural needs?
3. In connecting Mrs Malik's needs as cultural, does this then ignore that all humans are cultural beings, thus seeing people of different ethnicities as exotic/different?

Write your thoughts here

_____

_____

_____

_____

_____

_____

_____

Some things you may have considered from the above case study:

- Why do you think the staff felt that Sue's need for having visitors was less important than Mrs Malik's? If the dimensions of culture and cultural care are defined only by ethnicity or race, then it is more likely that your practice of culturally competent care narrows. This affects equity of care and you can also end up ignoring the needs of some patients.

- In denying Sue some comfort in a personally challenging time, what are Sue's cultural needs? Sue's cultural needs now, as a palliative care patient, could be based around needing some comfort from her family (and for them as well), at a very difficult time, as she copes with her grief. Culture, amongst other factors, are those things we each find provides us an identity and helps us make connections with those around us.

- In connecting Mrs Malik's needs as cultural, does this then ignore that all humans are cultural beings, thus seeing people of different ethnicities as exotic/different? Culture is more than festivals, religions, and ways of dressing that differs from the majority population. Not seeing all human behaviour as cultural to a point is to ignore the need for person-centred care, because you think that, as they look like you, their needs are the same. A culturally competent Registered Nurse provides care to all patients by treating them as individuals.

INTERCULTURAL COMMUNICATION APPREHENSION

There is a concept called Intercultural Communication Apprehension. Exploring this term may afford more insight into why sometimes: questions are not asked, enquiring about the patients preferences does not occur, stereotyping may happen or sometimes people may not even attempt to communicate with them. So, Intercultural Communication Apprehension is the fear or anxiety associated with either real or anticipated interaction with people from diverse groups, especially different cultural or ethnic groups. Sometimes, being overly 'politically correct' is also used as an excuse. We use the defences of 'not wanting to offend' as a way of avoiding conversations. An example of this is assuming a South Asian lady is Muslim and choosing a halal diet for her without checking on her preferences or not checking if an older White English lady may want a Caribbean meal for her lunch.

CULTURAL OTHERING AND EQUITY IN CARE

The nursing student should be able to appreciate equity in care delivery. This includes an appreciation of how all people naturally categorise groups of people as an 'other'. The practice of cultural othering is normal at one level. Josselson (2020) expresses that all of us construct a life story for every person that is met (consciously or unconsciously) within three minutes of meeting them.

From the moment a person is born, differences are learnt and recognised about what they are comfortable with. For example, learning from significant people in one's life includes how to navigate social situations. This includes attitudes towards individuals or groups of people (e.g. elderly, homeless, migrants). This kind of socialisation influences personal values which then predetermines how all of us interpret and act out professional values (Kinckle, 2020). The way those patients whose values may differ from the main way of seeing the world is more likely to reflect what was learnt as a child or young adults. For the nursing student who is not self-aware, there can be a lack of congruence between the way they behave, their attitude, the way they verbally communicate with those patients, and their opinion of them. For example, anxiety and avoidance of patients who present within the Emergency Department, who have a mental health diagnosis, can be related to those pre-judgements absorbed from the media on how they might behave or try to harm another person.

Categorising groups of people as an 'other' can also lead to stereotyping. Stereotypes are a psychological defence tool that is used to organise and categorise information about the numerous groups of people in society (Berry et al., 2011). Branscombe and Baron (2017) define stereotypes as the belief and expectation about what members of other groups are like. When stereotyping takes place, generalisations are made and this information allows predictions about the behaviour of that group's members to be made before it happens. Stereotyping becomes a problem when overgeneralisations and beliefs that all members of a group share the same attitudes, values, or behaviours. Any failure or deviance witnessed is attributed to as a characteristic of the whole group, homogenising them. Stereotypes are often inaccurate representations of a person or a group and, importantly, deny the uniqueness of individuals (Berry et al., 2011).

> *My father always said to me, 'A person's name is their most important possession. Never get it wrong.' That principle has opened up so many relationships to me... I treat other people as persons, not as instruments. And that leads to their treating me likewise.*
>
> **– John Thompson in an email to The Current**

The above quote is taken from an online article – consider the importance of how to navigate the area of diverse names (CBC Radio, 2016).

CASE STUDY

A new patient was admitted over the weekend onto a gynaecological ward. Her name has only just been listed on the board behind the patient's bed. The name says Pratixsha. Precious is a Registered Nurse and is unsure about how to pronounce this patient's name. She doesn't want to offend the patient by saying it incorrectly, so she avoids saying her name altogether. Precious notices that her colleagues do the same. Precious and her colleagues provide the same high level of care for Pratixsha as they do with all the other patients on the ward. However, Pratixsha has noticed that the staff avoid ever referring to her by her name.

Consider:

You are admitted into a ward for your care.

1. How would you like to be addressed by the people that care for you?
2. If an individual does not know your name, or your name is unusual, what would you deem as a respectable way of finding out?
3. What do you think would happen if you mispronounce the patient's name or ask them how to pronounce it?

Write your thoughts here

_____

_____

_____

_____

_____

_____

_____

You may have considered how a patient experiences their care and what makes you feel comfortable and uncomfortable with it and how this can be addressed. Often the best way to approach someone whose name you cannot pronounce is to try saying it and say, 'I hope I got that right?'. Commonly, other than Western names and some Gaelic names, most names are phonetic. Even asking a person how to pronounce it would be acceptable, instead of avoiding, or renaming them to make your life easier.

CASE STUDY

James is a 33-year-old Orthodox Jewish man from Manchester who has been admitted to your unit. He was diagnosed with bipolar disorder about 10 years ago. He has been an in-patient on your unit twice, in the past three years. The staff have reported that he does not mix nor engage in any of the available activities. He does not participate in the available activities such as playing snooker, playing puzzles, or watching television. Instead, he spends his time by his bed, reading from his religious texts.

The Registered Nurse from the night shift says he often finds James in the early hours of the morning 'rocking back and forth' while muttering to himself. Because of this report his medication for his agitation has been increased.

CASE STUDY—cont'd

You are James' named nurse and James' father Mr Drew comes to visit. Your discussion with Mr Drew does not go well, as his son appears more drowsy than normal. When you explain what has been happening Mr Drew becomes very angry. He explains that the 'rocking' is a normal part of the way in which Jewish people pray. Also, in his community people do not engage in activities such as games nor watch television. They mainly spend the day reading and engaging with their religious practices and culture.

Consider:

1. Where could the team or you have accessed information about the religious and cultural practices of James' Orthodox Jewish group?
2. Mr Drew states that the staff must stop comparing all religions and cultures to the practices of Christianity and the practices of the White majority population. What are the risks for all levels of Registered Nurses to be stereotyping in this way?
3. It is inevitable that we perceive other cultures and religions from our own understanding/lens. For example, there are several different Orthodox Jewish communities within Manchester. How would you find out what James' practices are?

Write your thoughts here

_____

_____

_____

_____

_____

_____

_____

Points for consideration:

- You could have asked the patient, his family, or your local synagogue or looked for information from a trusted source on the internet.
- Often Abrahamic religions (Islam, Christianity, and Judaism) have similar ways of worship, but culturally, dependant on where their ancestors are from, this changes. People can be insensitive when asking patients or friends from different backgrounds questions such as, 'When is your Christmas?' or 'What is your main religious text?' when other religions may not have anything similar to compare it to.
- As the first question in this section, ask James, or his family. Do not avoid asking questions in an attempt to 'avoid offending'. It would be worse to stereotype or, as in the case of James, cause him more harm.

Watch the Ted Talk (2009) The danger of a single story by Chimamanda Ngozi Adichie

Note your responses to this video in the context of this chapter. What were the take-home messages for you?

Write your thoughts here

_____

_____

_____

_____

_____

_____

_____

BEING AN ALLY

An ally is an advocate who supports and presents the patient's point of view or perspective in a situation where they cannot do this for themselves. The ally is willing to hear the story of the patient, who empathises with the patient and who ensures that the patient's voice is heard or that they are not discriminated against by those who have a professional responsibility to care for them.

Being an ally and challenging discrimination can be difficult. Becoming self-aware and developing the skills of a culturally competent nursing student is not straightforward as it requires people to consider previous behaviours and requires self-introspection.

There may be apparent forms of discrimination and micro-aggressions such as overt and covert discrimination, verbal abuse, insults, inappropriate jokes, ridicule, coersion, isolation, power play, and inappropriate or outdated language that is witnessed, sometimes reduced to 'I am just joking' when hurt is expressed. These kinds of behaviours and structural discriminators are often invisible to those in power and can be entrenched in the culture of nursing and within society. They can sneak up on both the victims and in our own minds and mouths, without us being aware. People working alongside may not notice it because 'it is just the way we work' or 'she's always like that but she's a great nurse'.

Search the internet for what the term 'micro-aggressions' mean. Look in the 'images' section of your search to strengthen your understanding of this.

What would or could you do if you witnessed micro-aggressions towards a colleague or patient when in practice?

Write your thoughts here

_____

_____

_____

_____

_____

_____

_____

Challenging discriminatory behaviour or micro-aggressions by a staff member as a nursing student can present difficulties, as most nursing students may not believe they have the social power or authority to challenge the behaviour of others. Watch How microaggressions are like mosquito bites: same difference on YouTube (Fusion Comedy, 2016) for you to really understand the concept.

If you are confronted by or are a witness to a colleague or patient who is displaying discriminatory behaviours or language, it is imperative to think before acting. Think about the scenario and each person as a unique situation. The culturally competent nursing student could approach these situations in a number of ways:

 TIP

Instead of directly saying, 'You are wrong', you could simply say, 'I am surprised, that's not my experience, and it's not the experience of our other colleagues'.

TIP

You could also use more neutral ways of challenging micro-aggressions such as: 'I've found if you do it this way/experienced the opposite.../Some people would tell you.../I'm not sure that reflects my experiences.../I have felt differently when...'.

Other effective ways of confronting discriminatory behaviour include asking questions or suggesting neutral statements:

- 'Where have you heard that?'
- 'Have others said the same thing?'
- 'Have you talked to the rest of the team about this?'
- 'I wonder if the patient is having a difficult day because I did not have the same experience'.
- 'I suppose the patient is very anxious and we have to adapt to what we are doing, don't we?'

However, there will be occasions where discriminatory behaviour cannot be condoned.

NMC

THE CODE SAYS

'That those receiving care are treated with respect, that their rights are upheld and that any discriminatory attitudes and behaviours towards those receiving care are challenged'.

In this instance, the nursing student will need to inform the person in an appropriate manner as to why they disagree with what was said or done. It is important to remember that years of social conditioning are going to be reversed in one conversation. However, it is important, at the very least, to exert the expectations of our professional regulations regarding non-discriminatory practice. It is essential to remember that

Registered Nurses and nursing students can (and do) engage in micro-aggressions or discriminatory behaviour but it would be unacceptable to not challenge attitudes that can damage patients emotionally. Setting an example and challenging them can help create more honest communication and nuanced debate with those around. Even if these kinds of conversations can be sensitive and uncomfortable, it allows for the understanding of what are acceptable boundaries of culturally competent care.

A culturally competent nursing student will note that everyone will make mistakes in intercultural communication. It would be worse to then avoid and ignore such conversations rather than apologise and acknowledge that what was said was harmful to the other person. Instead, an approach of 'what could I have done/said?' would help re-establish the communication that occurred. Challenging inappropriate politically correct language as a way of avoiding questioning is central to this. Everybody has a role in improving everyone's awareness of equity, inclusivity, equality, and diversity.

CONCLUSION

Developing cultural competence is a process: an on-going evolution of learning, making mistakes, clarifying, and moving to a better understanding of the nuances of communication. It is not bound by any rigid rules of how communication must occur but through practise, patience, respect, compassion, and a genuine curiosity to learn from others.

Now, that you have finished this chapter. Make some notes on what you have learned.

_____

_____

_____

_____

_____

_____

_____

_____

_____

_____

_____

_____

_____

_____

_____

_____

_____

_____

_____

_____

_____

_____

_____

_____

REFERENCES

Beach, M. C., Saha, S., Park, J., Taylor, J., Drew, P., Plank, E., & Chee, B. (2021) Testimonial injustice: Linguistic bias in the medical records of black patients and women. Journal of General Internal Medicine, 36(6), 1708–1714.

Berry, J., Poortinga, Y., Breugelmans, S., Chasiotis, A., & Sam, D. (2011) Cross cultural psychology: Research and applications. 3rd ed., Cambridge: Cambridge University Press.

Branscombe, N. & Baron, R. (2017) Social psychology. 14th ed., Essex: Pearson Education Limited.

CBC Radio (2016) How Canadians can be more inclusive of diverse names. https://www.cbc.ca/radio/thecurrent/the-current-for-november-24-2016-1.3864332/how-canadians-can-be-more-inclusive-of-diverse-names-1.3864356

Clarke, K. A., Barnes, M., & Ross, D. (2018) I had no other option: Women, electroconvulsive therapy, and informed consent. International Journal of Mental Health Nursing, 27(3), 1077–1085.

Cultural Intelligence Center (2020) Unconscious bias training without CQ makes things worse. https://culturalq.com/blog/unconscious-bias-training-without-cq-makes-things-worse/

Francis, G.(2009) Developing the cultural competence of health professionals working with Gypsy Travellers. Mary Seacole Award. http://www.gypsy-traveller.org/wp-content/uploads/2010/08/Gill-Francis-Cultural-Competence-Gypsy-Traveller-MS-Project-Report-2010.pdf

Fusion Comedy (2016) How microaggressions are like mosquito bites: Same difference. https://www.youtube.com/watch?v=hDd3bzA7450

Garcia, M., Mulvagh, S.L., Noel Bairey Merz, C., Buring, J.E. and Manson, J.E. (2016) Cardiovascular disease in women, clinical perspectives. Circulation Research, 118, 1273–1293.

Helman, C. (2007) Culture, health and illness. CRC Press. London.

Josselson, R. (2020) Narrative and cultural humility: Reflections from 'the Good Witch' teaching psychotherapy in China. Oxford University Press. New York.

Kinckle, S.R. (2020) Unconscious bias training without CQ makes things worse. https://culturalq.com/blog/unconscious-bias-training-without-cq-makes-things-worse/

Lloyd, B., Blazely, A., & Phillips, L. (2018). Stigma towards individuals who self harm: Impact of gender and disclosure. Journal of Public Mental Health, 17(4), 184–194. https://doi.org/10.1108/JPMH-02-2018-0016

Nursing and Midwifery Council (2018) The Code: Professional standards of practice and behaviour for nurses, midwives and nursing associates.

Papadopoulos, I. (2006) The Papadopoulos, Tilki and Taylor model of developing cultural competence. Transcultural health and social care: Development of culturally competent practitioners, 7–24.

Papadopoulos, I. (2018) Culturally competent compassion. Oxon: Routledge.

RCN (2011) Spirituality in nursing care: A pocket guide. https://www.elament.org.uk/media/1205/spirituality_in_nursing_care-_rcn_pocket_guide.pdf

RCN (2019) Legal update: Expressing religious beliefs. *RCN Magazines*. https://www.rcn.org.uk/magazines/activate/2019/oct/legal-update-religious-beliefs-in-the-workplace-oct-2019

Ted Talk (2009) *Chimamanda Ngozi Adichie: The danger of a single story*. https://www.youtube.com/watch?v=D9Ihs241zeg&t=594s

Volmert, A., Gerstein Pineau, M., & Kendall-Taylor, N. (2016) *Talking about poverty: How experts and the public understand UK poverty*. https://www.jrf.org.uk/report/talking-about-poverty-how-experts-and-public-understand-uk-poverty

Walker, E. (2019) What should co-production in health look like? *UCL Partners*. https://uclpartners.com/blog-post/co-production-health-look-like/

Weissman, J.S., Millenson, M. L., & Haring, R. S. (2017). Patient-centered care: Turning the rhetoric into reality. The American Journal of Managed Care, 23(1), e31–e32.

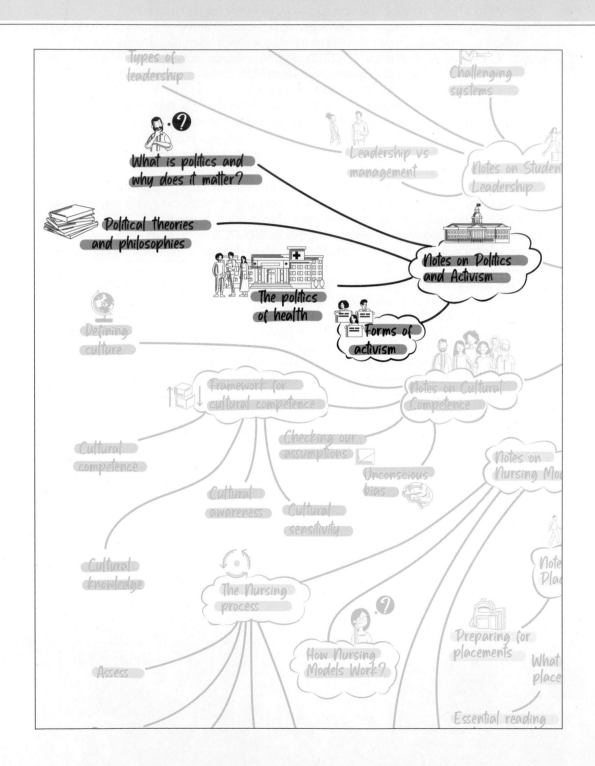

Types of leadership

Challenging systems

What is politics and why does it matter?

Leadership vs management

Notes on Student Leadership

Political theories and philosophies

Notes on Politics and Activism

The politics of health

Forms of activism

Defining culture

Framework for cultural competence

Notes on Cultural Competence

Cultural competence

Checking our assumptions

Unconscious bias

Notes on Nursing Mo...

Cultural awareness

Cultural sensitivity

Cultural knowledge

The Nursing process

Note... Plac...

How Nursing Models Work?

Preparing for placements

What place...

Assess

Essential reading

NOTES ON POLITICS AND ACTIVISM

Stuart Tuckwood (He/Him)

INTRODUCTION

Ahead of you there are 2,300 hours of placement, 2,300 hours of nursing theory, many more hours of home study, a part-time job, no doubt, and quite rightly some attempts to enjoy yourself, to keep your sanity and see your family. You'll be forgiven then for wondering why you should bother, as a nursing student, to read a chapter of a textbook about politics and activism. Many students and nurses go quite happily through their whole careers without caring at all about politics.

Unfortunately, politics does matter a whole lot to you and your future. It matters because of your tuition fees, your financial support, the childcare for your kids, the NHS, and the amount you'll earn for the rest of your career.

TWEET
@CharlotteNHSRN:

'Being politically engaged as nurses enables us to be better advocates for our patients and for social justice, a core value of the nursing profession'

TWEET

@AnnGregoryRN:

'It's the politicians who decide how much money the #NHS gets, and where it's used (unfortunately /usually / therefore we have to be interested. Think - who makes the decision about bursaries)'

Politics underpins the economy and our wellbeing. It's true that many nurses do not care hugely about politics, but many nurse leaders have gone on to become politicians or to have influence over political events. This chapter provides a brief insight into the world of politics and activism. It aims to convince you both that politics is important and that you have a valid voice and opportunity to become an activist who influences events.

You'll learn about some of the key political schools of thought and consider the recent political history of the UK and how it has affected your career and the health and wellbeing of the people you will care for. Several political nurses will give their perspectives on politics and activism and why you should care deeply about more than your day-to-day role.

Politics is a subjective matter, so you may not agree with the opinions and perspectives included as the chapter progresses. That is fine; debate and disagreement are necessary for politics and activism. Do not be put off, though; consider why you disagree and keep notes as you progress.

POLITICS IN ACTION

The decisions of those in power, based on their politics and ideologies, have a significant effect on your life and your future. Politicians make decisions, for example, about how healthcare professionals are trained and supported during their studies.

This was illustrated powerfully in England in 2016, when the Government decided to scrap the nursing bursary.

CASE STUDY

Previously, nursing students had received non-repayable financial support and didn't need to pay tuition fees for their courses. This change meant future nurses would graduate with many tens of thousands of pounds worth of debt.

The Conservative Party was in power in 2016. David Cameron was Prime Minister and Jeremy Hunt the Health Secretary. The Conservatives had been the biggest party in a coalition with the Liberal Democrats for the previous 5 years, during which time they had implemented a programme of austerity, cutting public services with the justification of reducing Government debt.

The Government argued that these students would earn graduate salaries in future and so should contribute to their training through tuition fees.

Critics argued that the move would deter students from nursing at a time when the UK faced a huge nursing shortage. They also pointed out that student nurses care for patients whilst on placements and that it was unethical to put them into debt while they did this.

Do you agree or disagree with this decision? Make some notes to support your opinion. If you disagree, what would you have done about it? How could you have tried to influence the Government?

_____

_____

_____

_____

_____

_____

This programme of 'austerity' had been deeply controversial. Freezing welfare payments, for example, meant that poverty increased and restrictions to NHS budgets and cuts to social care meant the performance of the health service began to steadily deteriorate.

The decision to cut bursaries sparked outrage amongst nursing students, healthcare professionals, trade unions, and opposition political parties. Nursing students and their supporters marched in their thousands, having formed an attention-grabbing campaign called 'Bursary or Bust'. They were supported by trade unions which represented nursing students, including UNISON and the Royal College of Nursing.

Looking back it is obvious that this decision had significant repercussions for nurses and the NHS. Graduating nurses now begin their careers with more than £50,000 worth of debt. They will pay interest on this debt from early on in their careers and throughout their working lives, significantly reducing their incomes and standard of living.

The decision led to a significant decrease in the numbers choosing to study nursing and healthcare courses. There was a particularly big drop in the numbers of mature students making the decision to study these courses, depriving the profession of many who would have become excellent nurses. The shortage of registered nurses in the UK has worsened and staffing levels across the NHS and social care have deteriorated.

The Health Secretary, Jeremy Hunt MP, has gone on to become chair of the Select Committee on Health and Social Care in the House of Commons. In this role he has flagged the staffing problems affecting the NHS and has publicly acknowledged that not enough was done during his time in Government to tackle this problem. Though many have criticised the move there are no imminent plans to reverse the decision.

Reflect on the impact of this decision. Do you think students and nurses were justified in taking political action to oppose this move?

_____

_____

_____

_____

_____

_____

_____

POLITICAL THEORIES AND PHILOSOPHIES

Politics can often seem like simply a competition between warring political parties and personalities, a less interesting celebrity sideshow. It is true that people are often attracted to support or vote for a party because of a charismatic leader or local loyalties. Whether or not you liked his politics it was undeniable that Boris Johnson was supported by many because of his humour and charm. Many young people supported Jeremy Corbyn because they perceived him to be a principled leader.

Scratch under the surface, however, and competing political parties actually represent different political traditions with very different ways of viewing the world, power, economics, and society. These different philosophies and theories are often fluid and evolving. Their views of concepts like the state, society, or personal responsibility can be extremely different, with significant consequences for healthcare or our wellbeing. Public health interventions, as a specific example, depend upon Government funding and the regulation of society. Philosophical and political disagreements over the size and reach of the State are therefore key to their context. Many of the most successful health initiatives have been the fruit of positive relationships between scientists, politicians, and the state (Hunter, 2016).

Many books have been written on their different histories and theories which would be impossible even to reference in this short chapter. The following is a very concise outline of some of the key political traditions of our times, focused on the UK. Bear this in mind as you read and consider the different theories.

Free market, 'Laissez-faire' conservatism

In almost all modern, market-based societies there has been a contest between those who believe Governments should actively intervene in the economy and those who believe the economy should operate 'free' from intervention. Those who believe in 'free markets' believe the economy works most efficiently when free from Government intervention, with individuals and companies free to succeed or fail depending on their effectiveness and ability to earn.

Much of this tradition was inspired by Adam Smith, a Scottish economist known as the 'Father of Economics' who established the idea of the 'invisible hand' of the market. 'Laissez-faire' is a French term which loosely translates as 'let free'.

Other key thinkers who perpetuated this tradition in more modern times were Milton Friedman and Friedrich Hayek.

This approach to managing societies has been in the ascendancy for much of the recent past as the world economy has become globalised. In the UK this tradition is most closely followed by the Conservative Party but there are believers in other parties also.

Margaret Thatcher took an aggressively free-market approach during her time as Prime Minister in the 1980s which meant many previously state-owned companies were privatised, domestic industries like shipbuilding and coal mining were allowed to decline, and the size of the state was actively reduced. Successive Governments have largely followed this tradition.

Socialism, communism, and social democracy

As societies around the world industrialised, much of their populations left rural agricultural work for factories and other heavy industries. Practices in many of these were often dangerous and oppressive, so the members of this new 'working class' began to organise to demand protections and better wages and conditions. Workers organised into 'Trade Unions' representing workers in their occupations but rapidly also joined with or formed political parties to further their interests. In the UK trade unions formed the Labour Party which began to compete seriously for votes and power in the early 1900s, entering Government for the first time in 1929 (New Statesman, archive 2022).

These working-class parties, to greater and lesser extents, were motivated by socialist, communist, and social democratic theories. These ideologies are more critical of free-market economies, believing that they lead to the exploitation of the working class and the further accumulation of wealth by the rich. Some of these movements and parties advocated immediate revolution to overthrow the existing societies to establish worker-controlled, socialist or communist Governments.

These groups often followed the theories of Karl Marx and Friedrich Engels, hence the term 'Marxist', and they seized control in many countries such as Russia, China, and Cuba. Other key socialist and communist thinkers included Rosa Luxemburg, Antonio Gramsci, and Lenin.

In other countries such parties attempted to gain power through democratic routes. In most places they gradually came to terms with capitalist market economies, though they support the greater redistribution of wealth and stronger public services and welfare. This form of 'social democracy' is strong in many parts of the world, but notably in Western Europe and Scandinavia.

The Labour Party has traditionally been the working class mass party of Great Britain, though its leanings have changed significantly at different time periods. More left-wing, explicitly revolutionary parties do exist in the UK but have had little electoral success.

Libertarian versus authoritarian approaches

Political leanings are often considered on a spectrum from the left (socialist) to the right (free market). This, however, only tells one part of the story. Another important consideration is the extent of individual freedom protected by different political traditions.

People with 'liberal' sympathies believe that individual freedom or 'liberty' should always be maximised. They will oppose restrictions on people's freedoms, for example, over their religious beliefs and sexual or lifestyle choices. 'Authoritarians' are more likely to favour interventions in people's personal lives. Many such Governments still prohibit homosexuality or prevent people from practising their religious beliefs.

Many extremely authoritarian regimes, like the Nazis and other fascist movements, have been in power at different times. The struggle between liberty and authoritarianism continues, however, even in supposedly modern democracies. The recent decision to remove women's right to access abortions in the US is a powerful example of this struggle.

Ecological and green movements

'Green' political movements have formed all around the world as concerns over climate change have risen in recent decades. Ecological and green parties have demanded actions to reduce harm to the planet, focusing on carbon emissions, deforestation, or air pollution. Though many have taken a long time to gain success, many have now begun to achieve significant support and influence. The Scottish Green Party is currently part of Government, as are the German Greens, and others have widespread support in Scandinavia.

Though some view environmental issues as non-political, climate change is increasingly being viewed as a structural and systemic injustice. Though the responsibility for human-driven climate change is driven primarily by the actions of richer, developed countries, the burden disproportionately falls on poorer people in developing nations. This means many green movements are assertively demanding the need for societal and economic changes to rectify this injustice and preserve the planet.

Liberation movements

Political movements almost everywhere largely shared one thing in common until recent times; they were almost entirely dominated by men. In Western nations they also largely excluded other groups on the basis of race or sexuality. Partly as a consequence these groups have experienced significant inequalities and disadvantages.

It was a long struggle in the UK before women achieved the right to vote, with campaigners such as the Suffragettes adopting militant tactics to force the decision. In many nations long campaigns of civil resistance and organisation were necessary to gain the vote and political rights for Black people and minority groups.

Significant inequalities between different groups still exist in every nation and political system. Liberation movements are those groups fighting and organising politically for greater equality. It would be impossible here to describe these in the necessary detail but some groups and campaigns of which you may have heard and could explore further include:

- *Black Lives Matter*. After the killing of George Floyd, a Black man in America, by the US police, there was an explosion in activism and protest against racial injustices and the oppression of people of colour. These spread around the world, including to the UK, and have led to a fresh questioning of why so much structural racism and discrimination persists in modern societies.
- *Feminism*. Feminist movements are those pressing for greater equality and rights for women. Whilst many people would think of famous historical feminist movements, such as the Suffragettes, who campaigned for political rights and representation for women, the struggle very much continues with women in many societies around the world still denied basic rights and equal opportunities.
  - Even in supposedly modern, liberal democracies such as the US there are political battles being fought over women's rights. The recent decision by the US Supreme Court to overturn *Roe vs Wade* and deny women the constitutional right to abortions is a stark example of this.

- *LGTBQ rights*. Until very recently, even in the UK and other Western nations, LGBTQ people such as homosexuals, lesbians, or bisexual or transgender people were denied many basic freedoms. It was only in 2014 that same-sex marriage, for example, was legalised in the UK. There are many active controversies still being fought around rights for LGBTQ people and many inequalities still exist.

An interesting example is that of 'Section 28', a regulation introduced by the Government which prohibited the *'promotion of homosexuality'* by schools in the UK. In effect this meant teachers couldn't actively discuss homosexuality which may have led many children to hide their true sexuality. A political campaign was fought against this regulation by those supporting LGBTQ rights and the regulation was repealed in the early 2000s.

'Before my career in nursing, I likely wouldn't have described myself as a feminist. As much as it pains me to admit, I was of the view that women's rights in the western world were more or less equal to those of men. Despite so much evidence of inequality, I didn't recognise the need for feminist politics or activism until I was nearly 30 years old. This isn't a particularly uncommon view, nor should it be surprising – it's a natural product of the ways in which women are socialised to see the things that happen to themselves and other women as isolated incidents. Without a feminist lens, it is harder to see how these experiences of inequality are part of a much larger pattern.

As a student mental health nurse, I quickly found myself up close with the stark realities of women's inequality and how it manifests in our communities and even within our own profession where male nurses progress faster and further despite comprising just 10% of registrants. Whilst it is true to say that both men and women can experience a variety of social, economic and political inequalities that contribute to mental and physical illness, for women these are layered on top of gendered inequality. In practice, this means that women are more likely to struggle with anxiety, depression and suicidal ideation. In

Scotland, women are also the fastest growing category in drug related deaths.

We might imagine that healthcare brings much needed balance when it comes to the care and treatment of mental and physical illness in women, but there are many areas in which women's outcomes are worse simply because they are female. Women's heart attacks and brain injuries, for example, are more likely to be missed by clinical staff than men's. One of the main reasons for this is that the majority of medical research utilises male participants, resulting in poor understanding of women's symptoms and with potentially lethal consequences. Unequal treatment for heart attacks alone contributed to the deaths of more than 8000 women over a 10 year period in the UK.

My interest in women's mental health led me to my current role where I support and co-ordinate care for victim-survivors of domestic abuse and sexual violence. Nurses can and should play a vital safeguarding role for these women and their children, since this type of abuse affects at least 1/3 of women and is the largest contributor to death, disease and disability in women aged 18-44. Nurses are, therefore, encountering victim-survivors regularly but many miss opportunities for intervention due to lack of training, confidence and resources.

These are common themes in health and why nursing and politics are so inextricably linked, whether we imagine ourselves to be politically inclined or not.

A good nurse recognises the political and social barriers to good health and wellbeing.

It is, therefore, just as important that nurses view women's health through a feminist lens in order to understand the additional barriers that stand in the way of women's health, wellbeing and equality.

Rudolf Virchow spoke of physicians as needing to intervene in political and social life and to remove the barriers to social functioning and good health. Without this, medicine cannot "accomplish its great task". As nurses, both before and after

Continued

registration, safe and effective care for women relies on understanding these barriers and intervening – in research, on wards, in communities and beyond'.

– Leanne Patrick, Gender-based violence nurse specialist

Nationalist Movements

There are many political movements around the world, including the UK, whose reason for existence is the promotion of a particular nationality or ethnic group. These are tricky to define as their philosophies and approaches differ greatly. Some were formed to fight colonial oppression and to exert their rights to self-determination whilst others more actively believe the groups they represent to be superior to others.

In the UK the Scottish National Party have been in power in Scotland for many years now, whilst in Wales Plaid Cymru enjoy significant support in many places. These two parties do not overtly express the superiority of their people, instead arguing for greater investment, localism, autonomy, and independence for their nations.

Reflect on the different political theories and traditions described above. Jot down how you think those who follow the different traditions might approach the following political issues.

- The funding and delivery of healthcare
- Public access to medical interventions such as abortion or contraceptive services
- Inequities in health between different population groups

_____

_____

_____

_____

_____

_____

_____

These answers are open to interpretation. Here are some thoughts you may have considered.

THE FUNDING AND DELIVERY OF HEALTHCARE

Those who believe in a '*free-market*' approach are likely to advocate for healthcare to be treated more like any other product. They view with more scepticism attempts by Government to intervene in healthcare and may oppose Government funding of health treatments and services. They argue that healthcare, like other markets, functions most effectively when individuals make their own choices about what services and treatments to purchase. This belief is more widespread, for example, in the US, where healthcare is largely privately provided and where individuals are mostly responsible for buying their own insurance.

Even in the US, however, the Government still funds and operates essential public medical services like Medicare and Medicaid. A huge political battle was waged in recent years when the Obama administration attempted to introduce a more active role for the Government in healthcare.

Those on the left, such as socialists, are more likely to believe that healthcare should not be left to the market. They argue that someone's eligibility for health services shouldn't depend on their private wealth and so they advocate that Governments should fund and provide essential care from taxation. This takes some choice away from individuals as the Government takes a proportion of people's incomes and chooses how to spend the money.

Socialists, under a Labour Government just after the Second World War, founded the UK NHS which to this day offers universal health coverage free at the point of care, funded by general taxation. However, you may be aware that moves in recent years by politicians are restricting Government healthcare funding and increasing the role of private companies. Accessing publicly funded services like NHS dentistry is becoming much harder.

Liberation movements often highlight how health services neglect the needs of disadvantaged groups. Feminists often point to evidence that women's health is neglected by the NHS in the UK, for example. They argue that health services should take a more proactive approach to tackling the inequalities which affect different groups.

Public access to medical interventions such as abortion or contraceptive services

More *liberal* political states tend to refrain from interfering in individuals' decisions about their sexual or reproductive health. *Authoritarian* Governments are more likely to regulate or restrict individual choice and autonomy over these types of decisions.

For example, in more liberal countries access to abortions is more likely to be protected. Access is restricted in many parts of the world because of this by governments which advocate 'traditional' values or which are wedded to particular religions. Many do not allow the operation of abortion clinics or services, denying women the ability to safely terminate a pregnancy.

Political movements of both the left and right can tend towards liberal or authoritarian approaches to these rights. Feminists and wider groups arguing for women's rights fight for funding and protected access to contraception and abortions.

In the UK, abortion was only decriminalised in Northern Ireland in 2019 and to date there is still no safe access to services. In the US many states are actively criminalising abortion following the recent Supreme Court Decision to overturn *Roe vs Wade*.

Inequities in health between different population groups

Wide inequities exist in health outcomes between different groups of people. The reasons for these are often described as the 'social determinants of health', which will be discussed later in the chapter.

Those who believe in the free market are more likely to advocate individual responsibility and opportunity, as discussed previously. They are likely to oppose attempts by the Government to intervene further in society to correct these inequities. They believe that in the long run people will become more prosperous if the market is left to operate free from interference.

Socialists and those on the left view health inequities differently, believing them to be a result of the imbalance of wealth and power in societies. They are more supportive of the Government intervening to reduce inequities between different groups.

In the UK in certain regions there are much greater levels of poverty and unemployment, causing worse health outcomes. The life expectancy of a boy born in Glasgow is more than 11 years less than that of a boy born in Westminster (ONS, 2020).

Nationalist movements often highlight these regional differences and may argue for more local autonomy, power, or investment to overcome them.

Governments can set up more intensive and proactive community health services in areas afflicted by inequalities to try to reduce them. Those on the left are more supportive of these attempts. But inequities between different groups don't just exist between rich and poor. There are serious inequities between men and women or between different ethnic groups, for example. Liberation movements have been highlighting these inequities for some time and argue for interventions to tackle them.

Research shows, for example, that Black women in the UK are four times more likely to die in childbirth than white women (MBBRACE-UK, 2021). Campaigners have been demanding that health services examine and take action to dismantle these systemic inequities.

The politics of health

Hopefully your reflections made you think about the different ways health and healthcare can be viewed depending on where you stand politically. In the UK we often take the NHS and universal healthcare as a given but in reality it is a politically contested choice to provide this.

In the following quote Ann Keen, a nurse, former Member of Parliament, and Health Minister, explains how nursing and health led her into a career in politics (Fig 8.1).

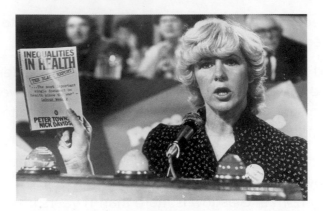

Figure 8.1   Ann Keen, Former Member of Parliament and Health.

'I remember that I had requested a late shift as I had been working the night before the General Election of 1979. Margaret Thatcher was elected Prime Minister. On my first day as a Staff Nurse, to my horror, as I introduced myself to the patients I saw many had portable TV on their locker and I saw our new Prime Minister waving as she entered number 10.

I chose a career in District Nursing. As a Sister in the 1980s I was made very aware of the poverty of the people I visited, in particular during the colder months. I recall visiting older frail patients with crumbling hips or cataracts. My patients were often generally unwell and very cold, living in one room alone in pain and cold.

It was not unusual for me to see my breath in the house as I was visiting. I constantly asked "please put your heating on, let's try to get you warmer" and the answer always was, "oh nurse if only I could afford to, I only have some money put by for my funeral, never mind I will be OK."

My heart would break, knowing that this was a political decision. I was angry as there was no heating allowance, our state pensions were the lowest in Europe, there was no assistance and no one in the Government seemed to care. During one visit I entered a house that was freezing. I was so cold myself and in this little room I found Annie, dead because of hypothermia. I cried and then had to look for a phone box to report this tragedy. Within a few days I discovered another frail elderly patient slowly dying again, so so cold.

As a nurse I could not provide heating, nutritional food or even good quality care, but I knew how to start the change that was needed. This made me decide to become more political and to stand for Parliament as an MP. It took 3 attempts, in 1987, 1992 and finally in 1997 when I eventually had the privilege of being elected to Parliament. I knew that this journey would now change lives. I was asked by Gordon Brown to be his Parliamentary Private Secretary, his political eyes and ears. I vividly remember sitting behind him when he announced that the Government would Increase the pension heating allowance and many other financial benefits. I thought of Annie and I had tears in my eyes. Do not tell me that all politicians are the same. I now feel sadly like we have travelled back to a time when a District Nurse, a Health Visitor or Community Midwife will be thinking, what can I do? I believe it is our duty to stand up and be counted whenever we see the terrible consequences of mean, harmful political decisions. We need to decide whose side we are on'.

– Ann Keen, Nursing advisor to Sir Keir Starmer, Leader of HM Opposition, former Labour MP & Health Minister, former Chair of Prime Minister's Commission Future of Nursing England

Ann's contribution illustrates why as nursing students and then nurses, you may wish to become involved in politics and activism.

Many of us became nurses because we want to support people to be healthy and to live fulfilling lives. Many soon recognise that there is only much we can do in our individual careers and through our clinical practice to support our patients, their families, and their communities. There are so many other factors that will influence their wellbeing and in many cases limit their opportunity to live healthy lives.

The Social Determinants of Health

We've grown quite used to lifestyle advice aimed at encouraging us to be a little healthier. We're told to eat our five daily portions of fruit and vegetables, to get regular exercise, and to watch our weight.

While these are all good recommendations, and it is important individuals take some responsibility for their own health and wellbeing, these choices are arguably less important than other factors largely beyond our control. People's individual lifestyle choices are also constrained by the wider social and economic conditions in which they live.

These factors are known as the social determinants of health, 'non-medical factors which influence health outcomes', in the words of the World Health Organization. Where we live; what we do; our level of education; our incomes; and our local environment are all factors which will influence our ability to stay healthy and live a long life, and there is only so much that health services can do to change these (Fig 8.2).

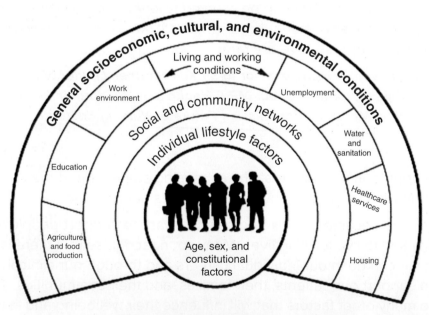

Figure 8.2   The social determinants of health, according to Dahlgren and Whitehead (1991). (https://www.gov.uk/government/publications/health-profile-for-england/chapter-6-social-determinants-of-health).

Simply put, the conditions of the society we live in affect our health and our life prospects in a variety of important ways (Marmot and Wilkinson, 2005).

When children grow up in cold, damp homes without the right nutrition, when the streets they play on are polluted and dangerous, when they face discrimination from the police or in the courtroom, and when they grow up and go to work that is poorly paid and demeaning, they are very unlikely to flourish and be healthy.

Expert, compassionate nurses, social workers, and teachers will have chances to support them and to open up opportunities but alone they cannot change the social determinants of health that hold individuals back and lead to health inequalities.

Politics and activism is the only way ultimately to change societies.

> *'Among professionals in public health, the political system is commonly viewed as a subway's third rail: avoid touching it, lest you get burned. Yet it is this third rail that provides power to the train...achieving public health goals depends on a sustained, constructive engagement between public health and political systems'.*
>
> *–Hunter (2016)*

The following timeline is an illustrative, not exhaustive, picture of some of the major political and economic changes since the year 1900 in the UK. Some of these are explicitly health decisions whilst others are related more indirectly.

This should give you an idea of why health depends so fundamentally on politics and make you consider why nurses might take a more active role politically.

As you read through the timeline, make notes on the impact you think these political changes will have had on the social determinants of health, comparing these to the suggestions.

_____

_____

_____

_____

_____

_____

_____

1900 – The Labour Party is formed, the first mass party of the working class in the UK.

The formation of a political party with the express aim of representing the working class supported trade unions in the improvement of working conditions in particular. Safer working conditions, better pay, longer rest periods, and weekends are examples of rights which were won by trade unions.

As working class people began to gain the vote, and the Labour Party began to win control in certain areas, public health priorities began to shift. More examination was undertaken of poverty, notably by Booth and Rowntree, and working class organisations made demands for jobs in civil works and improvements.

1908–1911 – The Liberal Chancellor Lloyd George aims to 'lift the shadow of the workhouse from the homes of the poor' by introducing the Old Age Pension Act.

For the first time those too old to work receive a guaranteed pension. In 1911 the National Insurance Act is introduced, which requires workers to pay national insurance, matched by contributions from the Government and their employer, in exchange for access to medicines and unemployment benefits.

The income from a pension, even if very low, will have affected many social determinants of health, including housing and living standards.

Though there was no NHS, the introduction of national insurance began the process of giving working people access to healthcare.

1914–1918 – The First World War. Britain fights with other Allied powers against the Axis countries including Germany and Austria. Huge changes occur at home as many women, still to achieve political representation, take up the jobs left by men joining battle.

At the war's end the 'Representation of the People's Act' gives the right to vote to all men over 21, and women over 30 who hold property. Women finally achieve equal voting rights in 1928.

The War, and the conditions it imposed on the UK population, had dramatic effects on many social determinants of health. Unemployment was reduced, for example, as all hands were needed for the war effort. Rationing was introduced in February 1918, which affected access to food.

The dramatically changing roles for women continued long-term changes in their education, employment, and living conditions. The ability to vote and engage more widely in community and political life meant significant changes to their communities and their participation in public life.

1929 – The US stock market crashes and brings a worldwide economic depression. Political and economic decisions in reaction in the UK result in more than 3 million unemployed people and widespread poverty.

The Great Depression, a result of changes in political and economic systems, caused much unemployment and changes to working. These of course will have led to changes in housing, working conditions, and diets.

1930 – A Labour minority Government passes the Housing Act, building on previous reforms on housing. This Act demands that local authorities clear slum housing and provides subsidies to assist in building more homes and rehousing families. More than 700,000 new homes are built as a result.

Slum housing promoted the transmission of infectious diseases and undermined people's health by forcing them to live in cold, damp, and unsanitary conditions. A mass improvement in housing standards obviously affected housing and led to improvements in life expectancy and reductions in many transmissible diseases.

1939–1945 – The Second World War. Huge social and economic changes occur on the 'Home Front' as a result of war. Heavy industry is devoted to the war effort. Food and other necessities are rationed, which continues for a long period after the war. Many are conscripted to fight the fascist powers of Germany, Italy, and Japan.

Rationing again affected people's access to food, though in many places the equality of this meant some families actually improved their diets. Again huge changes occurred in working conditions and employment as the war continued.

1945–1951 – A radical Labour Government wins the first post-war election. Many key figures played important roles during the war and now promised to use the powers of Government to tackle societal problems. There was a maturation of the welfare state and public health alongside this.

Many industries such as coal, steel, and rail are nationalised (brought under Government control). The National Insurance Act of 1946 establishes a much greater degree of social security. The National Health Service (NHS) is founded in 1948, offering universal healthcare, free at the point of use to all.

The improved and stronger welfare state protected people from poverty and poor living conditions if they were sick or unemployed.

The NHS, as it evolved and grew, offered access to healthcare services for all, meaning millions who otherwise would have been unable to afford treatment were cared for.

Almost more than any other, this period demonstrated the links between politics and public health. The philosophies of figures like Marx and Hegel had influenced the thinking of many politicians, notably Aneurin Bevan, the Welsh Labour MP and first UK minister of health.

Aneurin had been a trade unionist before becoming a politician and was highly influential in the founding of the NHS and our modern welfare state. (Hanlon et al. 2011)

1979–1990 – A Conservative Government under Margaret Thatcher allows the decline of UK heavy industries such as coal, steel, and shipbuilding.

Communities built around these industries in the north, the midlands, Wales, and Scotland see significant growth in unemployment and a loss of their traditional identities. The Government actively attacks the power of trade unions.

The decline of these major industries meant great increases in unemployment in many places. Cities like Glasgow, Liverpool, Manchester, Birmingham, and Sheffield, for example, were badly affected. Unemployment meant people lost their homes and incomes.

Less obviously, the loss of major employment in these industries deprived communities, cities, and towns of their identities and many of their social networks.

In many places social lives revolved around a workplace like a mine, a colliery, or a steelworks. Without these jobs and identities many were more isolated from their communities, a factor considered important in the poorer health seen in many of these places even to the present day.

1998 – The Labour Party, back in power from 1997, introduces the National Minimum Wage Act, for the first time establishing a minimum wage. This raises wages for the lowest paid in society.

At the same time the 'Sure Start' initiative is founded, which pours funding into interventions in the early years of children's lives, supporting parents and aiming to improve childcare, health, and education.

Improved wages meant better living conditions for many, allowing them to improve their living standards, their housing, and other factors such as their ability to engage in community life.

2006 – The Scottish Government implements a ban on smoking in enclosed public places, legislation which soon follows in other parts of the UK. The only members of the Scottish parliament to oppose are those of the Scottish Conservatives.

This political decision worked on an individual level, making it less likely that individuals would take the lifestyle decision to begin smoking. People's risk from second-hand 'passive' smoking was also reduced. As many people work in bars and restaurants this greatly improved their working conditions.

As you know, smoking is strongly negatively linked with many health conditions such as cancers and heart disease.

2008 – The Climate Change Act is passed by the House of Commons, establishing a legal duty on the Government to reduce the carbon emissions which are fuelling dangerous climate change.

It may be more difficult to see how this legislation influences people's health but climate change is the number one global threat to human health, according to the Lancet medical journal. Failing to act against climate change, which requires political and economic change, risks people's living conditions, access to food and water, working conditions, and many other determinants of health. By committing to reducing carbon emissions, the Government committed to acting to protect health also.

2010–2015 – Following the financial crisis of 2008–2009, a new Conservative and Liberal Democrat Government implement a harsh austerity programme which dramatically limits public spending.

Funding for social care in particular is cut back, the Sure Start programme is scaled down, and the NHS faces years of reduced investment. Pay for public service workers is restrained for a long period and the wider population sees wages stagnate for more than a decade.

Between 2010 and 2020 life expectancy stagnated in England and Wales and in many places got worse (Marmot, 2020). The austerity programme implemented by the Government affected the social determinants of health in many ways.

Wage stagnation and freezes on welfare meant many had poorer incomes, for example. Failures to increase housing supply meant many more living in bad housing conditions. The lack of investment in the NHS led to a serious decline in the quality and accessibility of health-care to the population.

2013 – Same-sex marriage is legalised in England and Wales.

Again it may be more difficult to consider how this decision influenced health. It is possible that the increased freedom experienced by same-sex couples by this decision enabled them to better engage in community and public life. Oppression and restrictions on freedom can cause people stress and diminish their mental and emotional well-being.

2020 – The Covid pandemic hits the UK, forcing the Government to implement strict lockdowns which limit people's freedoms in order to reduce transmission of the lethal disease.

The pandemic affected peoples living and working conditions, their education, and their access to health services, amongst many others.

The Covid pandemic is a prime example of how political decisions affect health. In the initial stages of transmission in the UK the Government insisted 'lockdowns' would not be an acceptable political move as they would overly limit individuals' freedoms. It is estimated that the delay in taking that decision may have led to tens of thousands of deaths (Ferguson, 2020).

On the other hand many have pointed out that lockdowns, and the disruption these entailed to social networks or access to health services, negatively affected the physical and mental health of people in many other ways.

Another consideration in this debate is that the UK public health system, enabling us to monitor and counter the spread of transmissible disease, was greatly weakened by funding cuts during the austerity period. This meant we were unable to effectively trace the virus and stop it from transmitting (BMA, 2020).

Now look back over the timeline. Select three of the political events. Note which political school of thought would have supported that decision and make some notes of those who would have opposed it. Consider why that would be.

_____

_____

_____

_____

_____

_____

_____

These are just some examples but you could have picked any from the list.

1908–1911 – The beginnings of the welfare state

Early attempts to make the State intervene more strongly in the welfare of individual citizens were resisted by those who believed in the free market. As Mullin puts it in a review of literature on the origins of the welfare state:

> 'A combination of the rise of trade unions, the founding of the Labour party and the extension of the franchise, along with a handful of enlightened employers and social reformers, forced social welfare on to the political agenda'.

1945 – The foundation of the NHS

The NHS was introduced by the Labour Party, during a period when there was stronger support for 'socialist' interventions like Government control of industries and more redistribution of wealth.

Naturally this was opposed by the Conservatives and others who believed in a 'free-market' approach. They did not believe the Government should take such an active role in healthcare or in industry.

2006 – The smoking ban

The debate over this political decision was more about the struggle between authoritarian and libertarian politics.

The move was broadly supported because the harm caused by smoking is so severe that most considered it reasonable for the Government to limit some individual freedoms to reduce it. This is particularly the case because many people who faced harm, such as bar or restaurant staff, had no choice but to go to work in these conditions.

In Scotland the legislation was opposed by the Conservatives. As you may have reasoned, those who believe the Government shouldn't limit individual freedoms opposed the move.

The Climate Change Act

This Act was introduced by a Labour Government but you may have noted that more widely actions to reduce carbon emissions and protect the planet are strongly supported by green political movements. Many of them felt this legislation did not go far enough.

You may have considered that forcing businesses and individuals to reduce their carbon emissions entails some amount of Government interference in the market.

This is correct and efforts to take more serious action to combat the climate emergency are still fought by those who strongly believe in a free market.

The 2020 Covid pandemic

The pandemic obviously brought further debates between left and right about the funding of public services and the NHS.

As you may have considered, however, the most controversial debates were between authoritarians and libertarians about the Government's powers to control individual freedom.

Should the Government have the right to force you to stay at home to reduce transmission of a lethal disease? Should they be able to mandate that you require a vaccination in order to access a public space like a library or a football stadium?

These are political debates with significant consequences for health which have no easy answer. Many nurses and other healthcare professionals have been vocally engaged in these debates on both sides.

What you think will depend on your political reasoning but it is certainly important that you are aware of the politics and motivations underpinning these debates.

KEY ACTORS IN POLITICS

In the UK, as in most other modern democracies, there are different branches of Government which hold different powers and responsibilities.

The three branches are the *Executive*, the *Legislative,* and the *Judiciary*.

The Executive

The executive is the section which implements policy, leads the Government, and conducts day-to-day Government business. Many modern democracies have directly elected Presidents whose office holds much of the executive power.

The UK is unusual in that the Executive is led by the Prime Minister, who is not directly elected to the position. The Prime Minister is an MP (Member of Parliament) and will be the leader of the political party or groupings which holds the most MP seats in a parliament after a general election, if they are able to form a governing majority.

The UK remains a monarchy with a royal family but in reality they have only a ceremonial role. The Prime Minister forms a Government after asking permission from the monarch to do so.

You may also have heard of the 'Cabinet'. This is not a piece of furniture; it is the group of the most senior Government ministers in the executive who meet to decide and enact Government policy. Senior Government position holders such as the Chancellor, the Home Secretary, the

Foreign Minister, and ministers with responsibilities such as Health all attend the Cabinet.

The Legislature

This is the part of the Government responsible for passing law. Many democracies have different chambers of law makers which serve different functions.

In the UK the MPs we elect sit in the House of Commons to represent their constituencies. This is mainly where legislation is introduced and voted on. Most legislation is put forward by MPs of the Government, enacting the programme they promised to voters before the election (though not always!). However, the Commons does have certain procedures through which individual MPs can put forward proposals to become law.

For example, MPs can introduce a '*Private Member's Bill*' calling for the law to be changed on a specific issue they care about. Most often these are not passed but occasionally the law has been changed by this route. For example, the Organ Donation Act of 2019, introduced by a Labour MP from Coventry, changed the law so that individuals are deemed to give consent to donating their organs unless they expressly opt out. This was a Private Member's Bill.

The UK second chamber is called the House of Lords. Second chambers in the legislature typically exist to offer balance and to scrutinise and improve legislation before it is finalised. In the UK the members of the House of Lords are appointed by the Executive arm of Government and they hold office for the rest of their life.

Traditionally the House of Lords contained many 'hereditary' peers who inherited their seat through their family and their privilege. Many of these have been withdrawn but to this day some still hold office, making the UK the only democracy in the world where a position in the legislature can be inherited as a birth-right.

The Judiciary

The judiciary is the third arm of Government. These are the courts and judges who interpret law and make decisions on what is lawful and unlawful.

You may think of judges and courts as only being involved in Ajudicating on issues of criminality but they have much wider functions. Elected Governments must still operate according to their country's constitution, if they have one, and to law.

This means that Governments can actually be taken to court to challenge their decisions and their policies.

An interesting example is the UK Government's recent decision to remove asylum seekers from the UK to Rwanda. Many people have challenged the legality of this policy and the first deportation flight from the UK was stopped when judges ruled it was unlawful.

Non-Government actors

Of course, you don't necessarily have to be an MP, a judge, or a Cabinet Minister to influence political decisions.

A wide range of organisations and individuals seek to influence political decisions on issues they care about or to promote their own private interests. These are some of the key ones to consider.

Trade unions. Trade unions are membership organisations that represent the members that pay to be a part of them. These members traditionally all came from the workers employed in a particular business or industry, though a number of large modern trade unions represent workers from across different workplaces and sectors.

Trade Unions use their collective strength to bargain with employers and bosses for better wages, terms, and conditions for their members. They often employ strikes and other forms of collective industrial action to force better deals for their members.

Many UK unions are expressly political and are affiliated to the Labour Party, which as we previously noted was founded by them. Others are not officially linked to Labour but will use their funds and influence to seek to influence politicians to further their aims.

The main Trade Unions representing student nurses, nurses, and healthcare workers are UNISON, the Royal College of Nursing, and UNITE. You should consider joining one during your studies.

Pressure groups, campaigning organisations, and charities. There are many, many pressure groups, campaigning organisations, and charities which set out to influence politics to address the causes they are concerned with.

Some will operate very publicly whilst others work behind closed doors to influence politicians.

You may be familiar with environmental charities such as Friends of the Earth or the Royal Society for the Protection of Birds. They will try to influence politicians by writing to them, briefing them on issues, or starting petitions. Often they will seek to get amendments or improvements to certain pieces of legislation which they believe are flawed.

Direct action groups. In any democracy the right to protest is a fundamental human right. Protest can take many forms, from signing a petition to attending a march or blocking the traffic on a motorway.

There is often debate in wider society about the extent of the freedom to disrupt the public through protest. Many campaigners believe the urgency of their cause provides their actions with legitimacy.

You may have followed the campaign of the environmental group 'Extinction Rebellion'. They have conducted attention-grabbing direct protests and disruption as they believe Governments are not taking serious action to prevent runaway climate change.

Some disagree with their tactics and believe they should be prevented from taking action. It is undeniable though that they have drawn attention to the urgency of the problem and protestors will point out that it was partly their action that caused the UK Government to declare a climate emergency.

Another interesting point to consider is that those considered extremists in their day are often later celebrated. The suffragettes, for example, conducted often violent protests against the exclusion of women. At the time they were considered by many to be dangerous terrorists, yet now they are seen as heroes.

Businesses and private donors. Those seeking influence for their private gain are also important to consider.

A vast range of businesses, commercial interests, think tanks, and lobby groups are always looking for opportunities to sway politicians towards their own interests.

In differing democracies there are varying degrees of opportunity for private interests to lobby politicians. Individuals or businesses may donate money to political campaigns or seek to sponsor events or meetings to get access to advance their cause. There have been many examples of corruption where politicians have asked questions, attempted to change laws, or placed donors in positions of power, when instead they should be representing the interests of those who elected them.

There is much concern about the role of private influence and money in politics. You only need to look at the eye-watering amounts of money raised by those campaigning to become the President of the US, for example. Many would argue that the need for such amounts of money excludes others from democratic debate and means the interests of the rich are put first.

GLOBAL POLITICS

Most of this chapter has focused on the politics of western democracies, such as the UK, the US, and most of Western Europe.

As nursing students and nurses, you should, however, be aware that many political and health issues are global in nature. Much of our food and products are imported from other countries, so we should be concerned with how they are grown or regulated; issues like climate change cannot be tackled by one nation alone.

You may therefore wish to research and look further into some of the global political organisations, bodies such as the UN (United Nations), which brings together all the nations on the planet to discuss and debate important global issues, for example.

The WHO (World Health Organization) is another you should consider. The WHO seeks to work internationally on global health issues, for example, by attempting to coordinate international efforts on communicable diseases such as Covid-19.

Though in many ways these organisations are supposed to be entirely fair and apolitical, in reality there is always politics at play and different actors seeking to advance their interests. The WHO, during the Covid-19 pandemic, for example, was accused from many different angles of protecting the interests of one nation over another.

ACTIVISM

Given the different forces at play and the money and power involved in politics it is easy to wonder, what can I do?

You may also wonder whether, as a nursing student and a soon-to-be nurse, you are able to take part in your activism, politics, and protest without risking your career and your job. As a nurse you will be registered and required to abide by the NMC Code. Though not registered when you are a student, your tutors will be monitoring your fitness to practise in future and any seriously unprofessional conduct could risk your future career.

NMC

THE CODE SAYS

20.7 'Make sure you do not express your personal beliefs (including political, religious or moral beliefs) to people in an inappropriate way'.

But what constitutes unprofessional conduct and what would be 'inappropriate?'

These questions are very debatable.

A registered nurse who became somewhat famous during the Covid pandemic, Kate Shemirani, was struck off the NMC register in 2021. She had attended many anti-vaccine and anti-lockdown protest marches and had given numerous speeches and interviews in which she made claims that Covid was a hoax and that vaccines were designed to kill people. The NMC found that she had undermined the reputation of the profession and contradicted public health guidance and removed her from the register.

This would appear to most people to be a clear-cut example of unprofessional conduct and expressing personal political beliefs inappropriately. But other examples are not so obvious.

In the early 2010s, as students across the UK were protesting against the introduction of much more expensive tuition fees, I intended to join in. I phoned the NMC to ask for advice on this issue.

How would they view it if a student nurse engaged in direct political protest and activism and ended up in trouble?

Unsurprisingly they wouldn't give me a direct answer to that question. I did go on to take part in marches, sit ins and occupations of university buildings in protest, being kettled by the police at various times. This made me feel uneasy and I was careful to ensure nothing I did could be construed as violent.

– Stuart Tuckwood, Registered Nurse

Being a nurse means you have a special responsibility, written into the professional code, to advocate on behalf of your patients.

NMC THE CODE SAYS

4 **'Act in the best interests of people at all times'.**

Some take that to mean that you should be vocal in protesting the social and economic conditions that undermine people's health, as proposed by Ann Keen earlier in this chapter. But many others would argue that being a nurse doesn't necessarily mean you should take up this role and there is certainly no political consensus across the profession. Some would argue that nurses should fundamentally be apolitical.

Another section of the NMC Code requires you to care for your patients regardless of their characteristics or views.

NMC

THE CODE SAYS

1 'You make sure that those receiving care are treated with respect, that their rights are upheld and that any discriminatory attitudes and behaviours towards those receiving care are challenged'.

Unquestionably, during your career you will have to care for people you dislike or disagree with. It would be seriously unprofessional for you to advocate your political views if it caused discomfort or offence to someone you were caring for.

This debate is far from clear cut, so there is no easy answer to this question of nursing and activism. However, becoming a nurse means becoming an expert healthcare professional, able to assess situations and exercise professional judgement. You should apply this same judgement in your personal life.

Would you attend a march in support of a political movement with openly racist or homophobic views? Doing that could reasonably lead people to question your ability to care properly for gay people or people of different races.

Would you occupy the premises of a fossil fuel company with Extinction Rebellion to protest dangerous climate change? Many doctors and nurses are undertaking direction action like this, believing their actions to be justifiable in the face of such a threat.

The decision ultimately has to be yours, but you should certainly consider your actions carefully and how they appear to others.

Even if you wouldn't engage in politics 'on the streets', there are many other ways to influence politics, healthcare, and wider society beyond just your day-to-day nursing role.

We make progress as a society on many issues because people are able to do this professionally. In many areas of nursing there is great debate about politics, advocacy, and topical issues, in which you can become involved. Nursing academics, for example, are constantly debating and arguing and critiquing each other on the issues of the day. That is part of being a professional.

> *'If we want to understand policies and outcomes, we need a more sophisticated understanding of political systems and institutions that shape the political processes and conditions for policy adoption'*

> **—Greer et al. 2017 argue in fact that an understanding of the realities of political systems and institutions is crucial for those who want to improve public health.**

Here are a few of the ways you might consider influencing politics and others during your career.

Publishing and writing

During your undergraduate studies it may be at times that nothing is further from your mind than writing and publishing your own opinion on nursing issues!

But great opportunities do exist for you to write and contribute to professional debates and discussions. Though you may lack experience or the specialist knowledge of many of your qualified nursing colleagues, your opinion does matter and you will have something different or important to say.

Some nursing publications such as the *Nursing Times* and *Nursing Standard* have spots for student contributors and editors. You could also contribute by reviewing other articles and submissions. It may be that during your studies you could also contribute to some research studies, for which you could contribute to the publication.

Activism and political action

There will be many societies, charities, and campaigning organisations at your university in which you could become involved. Think about what issues you care about and where you feel your energy could make a difference. Getting involved in student campaigning or charity work also shows potential future employers that you're caring and committed. You'll definitely learn lots from the people you meet and interact with.

You could also become a member of a political party and consider volunteering to support them locally. I've knocked on thousands of doors to deliver leaflets and campaign in elections and whilst it can be intimidating at first, it helps to build confidence and can be very inspiring when you meet like-minded people or have some success.

Often these parties will have other opportunities to volunteer which you might be interested in. You could support an MP to respond to local issues, for example, or assist members of the party in action to help a local charity or protect a local space.

Trade unions and professional bodies

Trade unions, described earlier in the chapter, are also an exciting way to influence your profession and wider society. You need to join a trade union as a member before you can get involved, but you should strongly consider doing this anyway for the personal representation and benefits you receive.

Unions are democratic organisations, so as a member you will get the opportunity to vote for the leaders who take up elected positions and also on the union's policies.

Trade unions also hold many conferences for their members to come together to debate and discuss their policies and plans. These are very exciting and there are normally fringe events and debates which you can attend as well. Unions are always keen to get younger and new people to their conferences, so ask how you can attend yours.

More broadly, trade unions and professional bodies are your professional voice. They represent their member's collective views and seek to influence society and your workplace to improve them on your behalf.

At the 2022 UNISON conference, for example, there were motions passed about tackling the sexual harassment of nurses and making international health worker recruitment more ethical.

Quote below, Mental health nurse academic and trade union activist Mick McKeown explains how he influences politics through his union and why you should think about this (Fig 8.3).

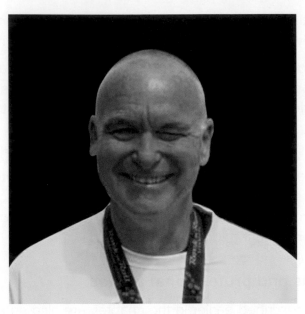

Figure 8.3   Mick McKeown.

'I have been lucky in my working life of nearly 40 years to have had a fruitful nursing career at the same time as being a union activist. I joined the union on my first day of work and became a representative soon after.

For me, joining the union was the right and natural thing to do and was strongly connected to an overriding interest in fairness – at work and in wider society.

Once I got involved, I consistently found opportunities for representing members in matters of discipline and grievance, and helping to build the organising strength of the movement, to be incredibly rewarding work. This also mirrored the fulfilment of my nursing role.

In many ways, being active in a union has been a complement to my personal and professional development, not least by furnishing a continuing stimulus for critical thinking, democratic cooperation and empathy for others.

At specific times my union has actively supported my career progression. For example, I attained my first degree as a mature student and received a small union grant to support my studies. This was a modest but telling launch of my eventual career turn into academia.

My choice of social studies was informed by my interest in matters of social justice, politics and economics led by my union activism but also supporting my growth as a critically engaged practitioner.

I have been fortunate to be involved in a very good local union branch supported by great comrades and leaders and to have had the privilege of serving for a long time on UNISON's national committee for nursing and midwifery.

After working in the NHS I am now a professor doing research and teaching in a university school of nursing. Along the way I have had grants from unions to do research into employment relations and union organising alongside my wider research focus into mental health.

This has involved very interesting work, nationally and internationally, addressing alliances between mental health service user/survivor movements, healthcare trade unions and critically minded professionals. Associated with this I have been involved in various campaigns and research focused on constructive critique and progressive reform of mental health services. This has been interwoven with union activism targeting broader social injustice and inequality.

As an academic, I have promoted the idea that activist and professional identities can and should be positively linked. I always encourage new student nurses and other colleagues to join a union and consider becoming active within it. In doing so, I can sincerely argue that my own career is evidence of the value of being active in a union.

Family and other inspirations were crucial in prompting my initial affinity for unions. My mum and dad were of the generation whose parents struggled for the founding of the welfare state. My mum, Sheila, was a nurse and midwife in the NHS and a supporter of unions.

My dad, Tom, was from a large family, all active within the union movement. He was a seafarer and then a car factory worker, becoming a shop steward at Ford in the turbulent 1970s; once helping to lead a nine week strike for an 18% pay rise.

Dock labour and seafaring had been the lifeblood of the Liverpool economy, and the communities which straddled the port were inextricably and intricately linked to their unions. Especially before the advent of the welfare state this was also bound up with strong social ties and mutual support in times of need. Once the NHS and wider state protections had been won, unions were crucial in defending these institutions.

Union density was high, and to be a union member was a valued part of worker and community identity. Arguably, present union organising concerns hark back to these times when people's connection to unions was understood more simply and passionately.

Our challenge today is to reconnect with those times when union legitimacy was not in question. Our organising task is made harder by a weakening of the connection between where people live and where they work. In our jobs as nurses, we can see for ourselves where the injustices are. We can also see that the unfairness that abounds in our modern society, exacerbated by years of austerity, unites nurses with our patients and service users.

These are at once trade union and professional concerns: union activism can be the flip side of a radical professionalism'.

– Mick McKeown, Mental Health Nurse Academic and Trade Union Activist

CONCLUSION

This chapter has aimed to give you a thought-provoking insight into the world of politics and activism.

For many people, politics seems like a world you'd rather avoid. It can be tedious, selfish, and angry, as well as seeming disconnected from your everyday life.

But politics is very relevant to your life and your future as a nurse. Your pay, the health of your patients, our climate, and the future of the NHS, all depend upon the decisions that will be taken by politicians and society in years to come.

We are still very fortunate to live in a democracy where you have a vote. But there are many more ways as an activist that you can influence politics. If you are passionate about something, which as a future nurse is highly likely, you should consider whether, through activism, you want to fight for it.

> *'If you fight you won't always win. But if you don't fight you will always lose'.*
>
> **– Bob Crow, RMT Trade Union, Ex-General Secretary**

Now, that you have finished this chapter. Make some notes on what you have learned.

_____

_____

_____

_____

_____

_____

_____

_____

_____

_____

_____

_____

_____

_____

_____

_____

_____

_____

_____

REFERENCES

British Medical Association, 2020. Austerity: COVID's Little Helper. https://www.bma.org.uk/news-and-opinion/austerity-covid-s-little-helper

Dahlgren, G, and Whitehead, M, 2021. The Dahlgren-Whitehead model of health determinants: 30 years on and still chasing rainbows. *Public Health*. https://www.sciencedirect.com/science/article/abs/pii/S003335062100336X

Ferguson, N, 2020. Coronavirus: Lockdown one week earlier could have halved UK's death toll, says Neil Ferguson. *Independent*. https://www.independent.co.uk/news/uk/politics/uk-lockdown-coronavirus-death-toll-neil-ferguson-a9559051.html

Greer SL, Bekker M, de Leeuw E, et al. Policy, politics and public health. *Eur J Public Health*. 2017;27(suppl_4):40-43. doi:10.1093/eurpub/ckx152

Hanlon P, Carlisle S, Hannah M, Reilly D, Lyon A. Making the case for a 'fifth wave' in public health. *Public Health*. 2011 Jan;125(1):30-36. doi: 10.1016/j.puhe.2010.09.004.

Hunter, Edward L. MA. Politics and Public Health—Engaging the Third Rail. *Journal of Public Health Management and Practice* 22(5):p 436-441, September/October 2016. doi:10.1097/PHH.0000000000000446

New Statesman Editorial, republished 2022. 3 August 1929: An Early Report Card for Ramsay MacDonald's Minority Labour Government. https://www.newstatesman.com/archive/2022/09/from-the-ns-archive-the-first-five-weeks

Marmot, M, 2020. Health Equity in England: The Marmot Review 10 Years On. https://www.health.org.uk/publications/reports/the-marmot-review-10-years-on

Marmot, M, Wilkinson, R, 2005. Social Determinants of Health. Oxford: Oxford University Press.

MBBRACE-UK, 2021. Saving Lives, Improving Mother's Care. https://www.npeu.ox.ac.uk/assets/downloads/mbrrace-uk/reports/maternal-report-2021/MBRRACE-UK_Maternal_Report_2021_-_Lay_Summary_v10.pdf

Office for National Statistics, 2021. Life expectancy for local areas of the UK: Between 2001 to 2003 and 2017 to 2019.

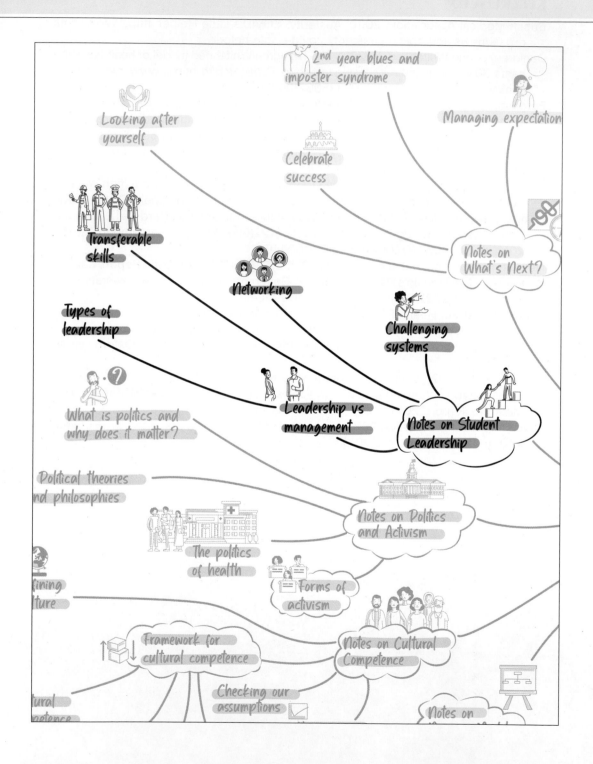

NOTES ON STUDENT LEADERSHIP

Paul Jebb (He/Him) ■ Heather Louise Massie (She/Her)

INTRODUCTION

Defining leadership and how it pertains to nursing can be closely linked to the nature of the nursing profession. Registered Nurses are constantly learning, adapting, and engaging in new practice (Mlambo, Silén, & McGrath, 2021), as indicated by the Nursing and Midwifery Council (NMC) Code of Conduct for Nurses (NMC, 2018). Registered Nurses have the professional responsibility to ensure they are promoting and providing evidence-based practice throughout all aspects of their work, and therefore Registered Nurses that influence positive change in a clinical area are often considered good leaders (Royal College of Nursing, 2022).

NMC

THE CODE SAYS

25 provide leadership to make sure people's wellbeing is protected and to improve their experiences of the health and care system

As a nursing student, you have the opportunity to witness many different leadership styles when you are rotating around different clinical areas. You will have the opportunity to witness multiple leadership styles in action, and the effects of this leadership on the team around them. You do not have to verbalise any of your observations but do consider reflecting upon them after your shift. Reflective practice is vital to us learning and developing as Registered Nurses (Patel & Metersky, 2022).

As a student, the notion of being a 'leader' can be quite an intimidating one. Some may be continuing a career path, fresh from college where necessary A Levels or similar qualifications have been undertaken. Others have decided later in life advancement in their chosen career or changing to a new career altogether. Already, nursing students come from such a massively diverse range of demographics, all with very different life experiences and approaches to challenges, which will be discussed later. Generally, the notion of leadership is tied to the premise of influencing a change within a clinical area (Tomey, 2008); but it is important for us to note that these changes are not necessarily large-scale changes. After all, our health service largely depends on every member of each team striving for high-quality patient care with each and every task they complete.

> **Take a few moments to think about how you feel about being a leader**
>
> _____
>
> _____
>
> _____
>
> _____
>
> _____
>
> _____

University is an interesting prospect. The level of academic rigour can be daunting to some and yet present an enjoyable challenge to many others. Looking at pre-registration nursing courses in particular: not only is the academic aspect an important thing to consider, but there is also the prospect of unpaid, full-time hours requirements during placements. Finding some level of balance between the two requirements on top of being able to work part-time alongside studies is vital, as the current funding doesn't quite extend far enough for most nursing students. These are quite significant challenges that should not be understated, so why the pressure on 'leadership'?

'As a first-year nursing student, I had worked in healthcare for 6 years. I still held the notion that leadership was something for senior nurses, management and matrons. It was something that could only truly be effective when defined by this specific group of nursing professionals, with clinical knowledge and experience far exceeding those around them. I did wonder why my university lecturers seemed so keen to ingratiate the thinking that anyone can be a leader, at any level. First-year passed in a blur; but I'd started absorbing the thinking that anyone can be a leader, even if I did so with a heavy dose of scepticism.

Here seems like a good point to note that I completed my studies while a national student representative within the Royal College of Nursing, which now seems like an incredible volte-face from my initially held views. This, to me, highlights one of the more important aspects of any person, not just a professional or a leader of any kind: the ability to take on new information, process it, and integrate it into cognition. If I had attended university to study nursing at the age of 18, I doubt I would have had this ability. Working in domiciliary care and then within the NHS as a healthcare assistant taught me humility, resilience, and the need to listen. In particular, the importance of simply listening cannot be understated, especially in nursing. But this also highlights how, especially as students, we all take different paths into nursing. Each pathway taken is rich in its own experiences, challenges that have been overcome, and knowledge gained'.

– Heather Massie, Registered Nurse

At the core of nursing practice lies the Nursing and Midwifery Council (NMC) Code of Conduct (NMC, 2018). Most frequently referred to as simply 'the Code', it breaks down the responsibilities of registered healthcare professionals – Registered Nurses, Midwives and Nursing Associates. The four main aspects of the Code are: prioritise people, practise effectively, preserve safety, and promote professionalism and trust. The NMC, as the nursing and midwifery regulator, is responsible for investigating any incidences where an individual on their registers may not have acted in accordance with this Code and determines their suitability to practise. It is worthwhile to read the Code, making note of any updates, but also to try and integrate the core aspects within your practice at an early stage; this will help you to create good nursing habits, and these will continue with you after university and into your career as a registrant. Revisiting it regularly and using the main aspects as the basis for your reflections when it comes to time to revalidate is recommended. Revalidation is a lengthy, in-depth process and getting into good habits of writing reflections early will make this process much simpler for you when that time comes. Throughout this chapter, there will be reference to the Code to demonstrate how these aspects can be drawn into your day-to-day practice.

LEADERSHIP AND MANAGEMENT

Leadership and management are two very different entities, but they are complementary roles. Managers are usually leaders of their areas, but leaders are not always managers (Valiga, 2019). A manager may rely on their senior clinical staff to direct staff and lead the team and to feed back to them. Sometimes this is under an official pathway but can be more informal. Managers sometimes underestimate their need for the feedback that these staff can provide, because it is often these leadership staff that have experienced a change on the 'ground level' and will provide the feedback to suggest amendments to ensure that the service continues to adapt positively. These unofficial leaders can provide a vital advocate for staff and the people who use the service, and the management. Strong, engaging, and inspiring role models for a team are vital to bringing success (Scully, 2015), in this case delivering the best quality of nursing. Bringing these separate aspects together under a shared goal is how teams continue to develop, improve, and adapt to changes under pressure. Strong leadership emphasises supporting staff and provision of high-quality support services for these staff, which gradually leads to the delivery of high-quality care, which is what we all intend to deliver as nursing professionals. Continuing delivery of high-quality care services improves the levels of patient satisfaction and therefore the overall public opinion of the service is likely to be much more positive.

The nursing profession has seen during the Covid-19 pandemic exactly how much stress the health service and the staff working within it have been under. These pressures are not sustainable for any kind of workforce, especially not one that works so especially hard each and every day.

Workforce wellbeing

As a leader and a manager, we must ensure the wellbeing of the teams we work in, lead, and work for. Leaders and managers have a responsibility to look after each other's health and wellbeing – physical and mental, as both areas can impact each other, which in turn, will impact our teams' working lives, ultimately affecting patient care.

The Covid-19 pandemic and other health service reviews including the Mid Staffordshire NHS Foundation Trust review (2013) and the Morecambe Bay Review (2015) have highlighted the increasing need for compassion and kindness within the workplace, and the impact this has on people's experiences of care – either across service delivery or the staff members own personal experiences working within the care environment. Compassionate leadership may be seen as soft and ineffective to leadership, but we need to show courage to be able to lead compassionately than to lead with command and control (West, 2021)

Staff experiences enhancing patients' experiences is a well-known concept, but an often ignored one and this doesn't happen. Staff are, at times, pushed to the limit of their emotional care due to operational demands and severe understaffing, as well as the day-to-day challenges people face in life. Leaders need to be able to recognise this and also role model wellbeing behaviours, taking regular breaks whilst at work, being able to access refreshments no matter what time of day, and ensuring their and others' annual leave is taken to enable people to recharge. This is all necessary to look after ourselves and enable people to rest and relax so that they can return to continue the work and deliver quality care to those who need it.

There are many different types of leaders, which some may already be familiar with. Each different type has its strengths and weaknesses, and it can take time to work out exactly which type of leader you are. A collective leadership culture can enable positive organisational change at the same time as promoting individual skill development for staff (Faculty of Medical Leadership and Management, 2015) which overall promotes an improved health service and increases the level of positive experiences for patients when they engage with the service. This thinking of collective leadership reflects the attitude that any staff member of any grade can create positive change if they wish to. The NHS Leadership Academy has a plethora of resources available to everyone, whatever level of your career. There are both bite-size learning resources and more in-depth courses; there are also leadership programmes that are tailored to different levels of staff. Anyone can develop leadership skills; you do not have to wait until you are thinking about a senior nurse or management role! If anything, developing this area of knowledge and experience at an early stage of your career can make future steps seem much less daunting than they can appear to be.

Although there are many different types of leaders, these can generally be categorised into five 'leadership styles' with advantages and disadvantages to each:

- **Authoritarian Leadership** – this type of leader will have clearly defined expectations of outcomes. This provides clear direction when the leader is the most knowledgeable individual in the team and is a useful approach to take when timescales are limited. However, occasionally this very strict style of leadership can lead to rebellious behaviours within the team, which undermines the overall outcomes. Due to the fact that team input is limited, creativity and innovative approaches are reduced, and this can have a negative effect on group collaboration (Fig 9.1).

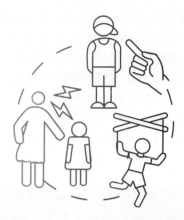

Figure 9.1   Authoritarian Style.

- **Participative Leadership** – this style of leadership focuses on the involvement of team members at all steps throughout the decision-making process, which can lead to an overall feeling of members of the team being more engaged with the project and more motivated to increase their overall level of input. However, this does mean that decision-making processes can become time consuming as ideas are put forward and discussed, and communication failures can occur if any decisions are not then clearly communicated in a set manner, which would leave them open to interpretation (Fig 9.2).

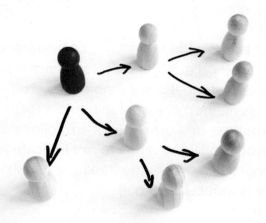

Figure 9.2   **Participative Leadership.**

- **Delegative Leadership** – you may have heard of this being described as '*laissez-faire*' leadership, which means tasks are distributed amongst team members and this then dictates how and when tasks are completed. This works well in a team of highly engaged individuals who can all work independently. However, in some teams this may not be appropriate, as disagreements between team members can lead to division in the group, which generates reduced morale (Fig 9.3).

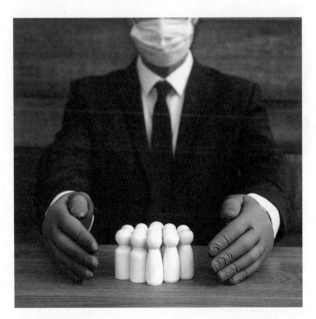

Figure 9.3   **Delegative Leadership.**

- **Transactional Leadership** – this style of leadership uses the notion of 'rewards' or 'punishments' to secure task completion. The leader sets their goals, and employees are rewarded for their input. This method of leadership has a focus on ensuring established routines and procedures are followed in already set manners of working, which tends to not indicate towards organisational change. Like with authoritarian leadership, innovation and creativity is reduced (Fig 9.4).

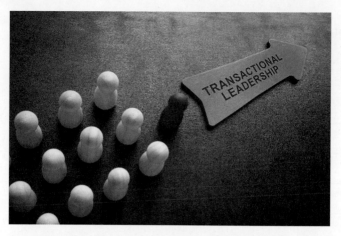

Figure 9.4   **Transactional Leadership.**

- **Transformational Leadership** – this type of leadership style seeks to inspire staff with what they aspire to achieve and then encourage and empower them to achieve these goals. It uses this motivation and inspirational approach to gain support from employees. In this manner of leadership, there is often perceived to be a high morale amongst the team. However, this type of leadership does require significant effort. Consistent approaches to motivation will keep the team on track and feedback sessions are extremely helpful in maintaining employee motivations (Fig 9.5).

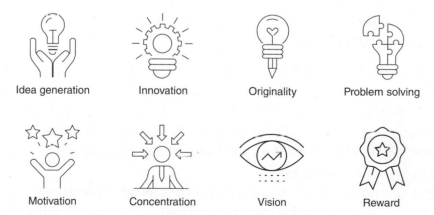

Figure 9.5   **Key elements of leadership.**

What leadership styles have you seen in action?

_____

_____

_____

_____

_____

_____

_____

The Healthcare Leadership Model

The NHS Leadership Academy has developed the Healthcare Leadership Model (NHS Leadership Academy, 2013), which outlines nine dimensions of leadership behaviour. These dimensions can be applied to whatever size of team or service you work within. It also highlights the importance of personal qualities, as the way we develop and manage ourselves often indicates how we'd manage others. Having a strong sense of self-awareness and self-discipline can keep us on track when trying to influence change within and improve any service. These dimensions are titled as follows:

- Inspiring shared purpose – valuing the ethos of the service and behaving in a way that reflects the shared values of the service
- Leading with care – understanding the unique qualities and needs of a team, and providing a safe, caring environment for staff to be able to do their jobs effectively and providing high-quality care for patients
- Evaluating information – seeking out new information, and effectively using this information to integrate new ways of working within existing models
- Connecting our service – understanding how the many different services provided all interlink within the larger health service

provision, and improving these links between services in order to provide seamless care for patients

- Sharing the vision – being able to effectively communicate aims for the future of the service and sharing in the planning phases to enable these aims to come to fruition
- Engaging the team – involving individuals in all phases and demonstrating that their contributions have had a positive effect on the continuing service delivery
- Holding to account – setting clear targets, supporting staff in taking responsibility for results and providing balanced feedback to staff, creating a mindset that enables positive change
- Developing capability – enabling staff to develop skills and attributes that will contribute to the long-term goals of the service development while also being a role model for personal development
- Influencing for results – understanding how to have a positive impact on people, building relationships across teams and with individuals to recognise their passions and their concerns, and using this to build collaboration across organisations

All these dimensions have a dual focus: provide support to staff and enable them, in turn, to provide a high standard of care. Of course, with the pressures the health service faces daily, this can be extremely difficult to do effectively. These dimensions can be embodied by any member of staff; you do not have to be an established leader to utilise them to develop your skills according to these dimensions. Simply implementing one dimension at a time into your daily practice will enable you to gradually develop your leadership skills (Fig 9.6).

The Healthcare Leadership Model is made up of nine behavioural dimensions:

- Inspiring shared purpose
- Leading with care
- Evaluating information
- Connecting our service
- Sharing the vision
- Engaging the team
- Holding to account
- Developing capability
- Influencing for results

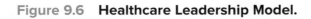

Figure 9.6   Healthcare Leadership Model.

Leaders also often take initiative. This can be the opportunity to demonstrate their abilities to be an effective leader. There are many ways in which some of us take initiative; in the way we approach our patients, the way we assist our colleagues in the completion of tasks, and ways in which we seek to create a more efficient and effective way of working.

'I was still a nursing student but had worked in the same clinical area for five years. As part of my role, I would inspect every space on the ward, checking the emergency equipment. For a few weeks, I had noticed that things like tubing were not cut to appropriate lengths, that the suction was not properly set up, or that things were missing. For those first few weeks, I would simply ensure that each space had the appropriate equipment and that any that required setting up, such as the suction canister, was properly done. I tried to explain to some colleagues about the problem and why we needed certain equipment in the spaces, but at this time I was only doing one regular shift a week, and therefore this limited the number of staff I could speak to. I decided to create a simple step-by-step manual that listed the equipment and necessary lengths of tubing, and how to correctly set up the suction canisters. I created checklists for each bay to act as a prompt for each member of staff to check the spaces as they met each patient. With the support of the Practice Development Sister for the ward, I created a quick video "how-to" to demonstrate how quickly this equipment could be set up, but also how vital it was to have this equipment ready in an emergency. The checklists and guide are still used on the unit today, as part of an induction and refresher package for staff.

The aims for my above actions were simple: patient safety was being compromised and I had the opportunity to implement a very small change that could improve safety and patient outcomes in emergencies. There was some negative feedback from some of the more-experienced staff, who felt that there was no need for such a checklist and learning, however the fact that our newer members of staff were not being shown effectively how to do this, which was having a detrimental effect on overall patient safety, I felt demonstrated that they were not able to take the time to sufficiently explain the need for this. I elected for the approach I did in order to avoid singling any member of staff out and made myself available for one-to-one demonstrations of equipment set up and explanations, which were taken up by some of the newer staff. I felt it was imperative to do as the nature of the unit we worked on often meant that we would have some extremely poorly patients, and therefore we needed to be able to access all equipment in a timely manner'

– Heather Massie, Registered Nurse

Transferable skills and necessary skills/behaviours of a leader

Increasing numbers of people commence their nursing degrees later in life. They may have already started a career in healthcare and be seeking to take those next steps. Others are changing career paths entirely. Nursing students from both areas may find that they already do possess skills that are vital to success in degree courses, and well into their careers. Some students come straight from college continuing their learning journey; their skills should also not be understated. However, it is frequently the case that nursing students are assumed to not have these skills and underlying knowledge. Upon completion of their studies and becoming a registrant, these skills are once again ignored by the system. This should not be an obstacle to you developing these skills early in your career and continuing to develop them throughout your working life. Use the skills you already have and use these in your daily practice, and you will see how you can develop while keeping in line with the Code.

What transferable leadership skills do you have?

_____

_____

_____

_____

_____

_____

_____

Registered Nurses and strong leaders have a lot of skills that match, even for those Registered Nurses who are relatively 'junior' staff or do not wish to pursue a management role, because many of these skills are encompassed in the wider understanding of the Code. Strong leaders should know how to appropriately delegate tasks, in order to ensure an overall goal is met. Registered Nurses do the same, to ensure all patient needs are met. Both Registered Nurses and strong leaders can prioritise their workloads, again to ensure that a larger goal is achieved in a logical manner. They are also able to constantly readjust their priority lists based on new information or changes to the situations around them at any given time. Registered Nurses and leaders must be on the mark with their time management skills, in order to ensure that all tasks are completed as and when they need to be.

In the beginning stages of your career as a nursing student and as a newly Registered Nurse, time management is a vital skill to master. However, even accepting this into our thinking, it is very easy as Registered Nurses for us to think, 'I'll just do this one task and then take a break'. Often, that one task becomes more and often leads to missed breaks. Taking rest periods during shifts is vital, and the fact that nursing is demanding of us should highlight this need all the more. As registrants, we make decisions that have a significant impact on our patients, and it is our professional responsibility to ensure that we are able to make these decisions (Linton & Koonmen, 2020). This means ensuring you are able to take your breaks and supporting the team around you to take their breaks as well.

Shift leaders, also known as the 'nurse in charge' or 'co-ordinators', often will try to mitigate any problems as they arise, demonstrating the necessary patience and flexibility that healthcare professionals must utilise when facing challenges to the ideal working process. In order to ensure that this is done effectively, staff should be consulted about the decision making and receive clearly communicated instructions on how these expectations are to be achieved. The staff should then be properly supported in order to deliver these goals, as much as is necessary. Some staff may require more support than others, and a strong leader should be able to recognise this, or at least be approachable for their colleagues to come to and ask for help.

These teams are often complex structures, encompassing a group of individuals of diverse backgrounds; varying levels of skills, knowledge, and experience; and different clinical responsibilities. Therefore, a leader should ensure that tasks are delegated appropriately, ensuring that high-quality patient care is always delivered, but also that the staff are supported in an effective manner.

Networking and relationship building

Professional relationships can sometimes be difficult to foster, especially outside of one's own Trust or organisation. However, finding links to other organisations can be extremely beneficial and worth the effort. Examples of implemented policies and procedures can be shared, and this shared experience can allow for ideas to further develop and, overall, provide maximum benefit to the patient. This is always key and demonstrates the effective implementation of one of the core aspects of the Code: prioritising people.

NMC

THE CODE SAYS

Prioritise People

You put the interests of people using or needing nursing or midwifery services first. You make their care and safety your main concern and make sure that their dignity is preserved and their needs are recognised, assessed and responded to. You make sure that those receiving care are treated with respect, that their rights are upheld and that any discriminatory attitudes and behaviours towards those receiving care are challenged

Social media is an inherently useful tool in developing these professional relationships. It allows for a partly professional, partly more personal link to another nursing professional, potentially in another Trust, or even in a different country. It allows professionals to share experiences of implemented changes, share learning, and overall improve the service that our patients receive. Sharing this knowledge and experience enables all patients, wherever they are, to be able to access a service that is suited to their needs.

Social media does, however, need to be used with caution. Professional disagreements can occur over any platform, but extra caution should be used on social media, or any public platform. The NMC has published social media guidelines (2019) and it is vital that these are followed, as these guidelines form part of the Code. Making contact with other students can enable you to develop an informal support network, as support is vital especially during your student and newly Registered Nurse years.

On a local level, seek out your union representatives, if you have a membership to one. Being a member of a nursing union is completely optional, and there are special offers for nursing students in terms of membership fees. These offers also may continue into your first year as a Registered Nurse. It is worth exploring the benefits of union membership, as there may be local and national events that look at learning that could be useful for Continuing Professional Development but also provide ample opportunities to grow your network of professional contacts. These events conveniently provide the opportunity to be in the same space as professionals with similar interests to you and often prompt group discussions.

These networking experiences also help to develop your own personal communication styles and identify where we could potentially improve. Using feedback from other professionals can help us to develop our approaches to achieving goals and working within teams, which in turn can lead to a development of leadership techniques. Occasionally, there are patterns that unfold in these events, especially if they tend to be attended by the same groups of people. You may find that there is an individual who takes charge of any group activity or someone who is able to create a good plan and organise the delegation of tasks well.

Effective delegation

Effective delegation allows for the transfer of accountability for a particular role or outcome and empowers staff to take clinical responsibility. It involves recognising the skills and talents within your team that enables the team to succeed overall, by focusing efforts on each team member's particular strengths. However, staff who have had a task delegated to them should not be afraid to ask for support and use it as an opportunity to develop skills that they may not feel entirely confident in. Task delegation is an opportunity to learn and develop but also to increase self-confidence. It also provides ample reflective practice opportunities which are useful for revalidation, and the continuing development of nursing practice.

Delegation is defined as the transfer to a competent individual or authority to perform a specific task in a specific situation (NMC).

THE CODE SAYS

11 be accountable for your decisions to delegate tasks and duties to other people

Delegation of tasks forms part of a Registered Nurse's role day in and day out. With the increasing development of support roles across health and social care as well as the development of the nursing associate role, effective delegation must be understood by practitioners as it is an essential component of safe quality care delivery and forms part of the NMC Code, which sets out the expectations of people on the professional register.

Delegation can be difficult and the registered practitioner must be able to delegate tasks safely. Understanding an individual's competency is essential, as well as clearly exploring the tasks, the boundaries, a need to understand the individual's understanding of what has been delegated to them, and also being able to ensure feedback is gained as reporting back following the delegation especially if there are any worries or concerns which may need future monitoring, assessment, or input from the Registered Nurse. Registered practitioners need to take responsibility for the delegation and be supporting those whom they have delegated to, and employers also have a responsibility to ensure staff are trained and supervised appropriately. Employers accept vicarious liability for their employees, meaning that people work within their sphere of competence and in conjunction with their employment, the employee is also accountable for their actions (RCN).

How do you feel about delegation?

_____

_____

_____

_____

_____

_____

_____

Developing our own skills as leaders

As previously stated, there are many different leadership styles which can influence how well a team functions in delivering an overall goal. Personal attributes largely dictate how well a person can lead a team or a service, but it is important that a period of strong performance does not encourage one to start being complacent in their leadership; a strong start will often eventually burn out, meaning a service will stagnate. It is vital that we recognise that there are always ways in which we can develop and improve, and within the NHS this is demonstrated by the appraisal process. While not entirely perfect, it does help staff to identify where they can develop new skills and improve existing ones.

In order to effectively develop and demonstrate leadership skills, especially while still a student, it is important that you are familiar with the policies within the Trust that you are working within and also how those policies are reflected on a much wider level. All local policies have a basis in national policy and standards. Understanding these and the local versions can help you to understand where there is room for positive change while still aligning with the existing policies.

Respecting your colleagues and your patients is paramount. We must acknowledge the contributions of the wider group of the multi-disciplinary team and take the opportunity to reflect on our own practice and consider the effects on the wider time. Remember: you are simply trying to do *your* best, keeping your standards of practice high and enabling other members of the team to also improve their practice. This in turn improves the standards of patient care, which is the overarching goal of any healthcare service.

How will you develop your leadership skills?

_____

_____

_____

_____

_____

_____

Equality, diversity, and inclusion

Equality. We know equality it governed by law, and employers have a legal responsibility to ensure that their staff all have equal opportunities to develop and progress through their careers. To deliver high-quality patient care, we must ensure every single member of our staff is supported appropriately. However, as is frequently reported, many of the systems in the UK healthcare sector routinely fall short of this. Evidence suggests that still, staff from Black and minority ethnic backgrounds are treated significantly less favourably than their White colleagues, and often have a poorer experience of working within the health service. A report from 2017 highlights that the health service cannot continue in this manner. This same report also stresses that this negative treatment of Black and minority ethnic staff has negative consequences for our patients (NHS England, 2017).

It is well documented across national media when patients experience inequality within the health service, and every time, there are apologies issued alongside promises to 'do better'. However, it is still happening. One regional review highlighted the race inequalities experienced by patients in their areas (Bradford District Care NHS Foundation Trust, 2016). This same report also explains that despite being aware of the ethnic diversity across the area, the workforce data suggests that these proportions were not reflected in the medical and nursing staffing within this area, with a disproportionately high number of staff from Black and ethnic minority groups facing disciplinary procedures, and a very low proportion of the Board members are from Black and ethnic minority backgrounds. Research suggests that patients from Black and ethnic minority groups report lower satisfaction with their care overall than their White British counterparts (Pinder, Ferguson, & Møller, 2016). This research also concludes that if healthcare providers and services had a better understanding of the needs of people from Black and ethnic minority backgrounds, then these patients may in fact have better overall care experiences and better outcomes.

Mentoring, reverse mentoring, and coaching

Part of the leadership role is to role model behaviours, as well as training and education and supervision of others; this includes developing people clinically, professionally, and personally. To do this effectively you will need to have developed your own communication skills to cover many situations. You will also need to be organised and proactive, work collaboratively with teams and/or individuals to agree shared goals, be assertive to agree shared goals, show your assertive skills to ensure you give constructive criticism, and also share your own knowledge of situations and potential solutions that you developed. Self-awareness is key, so you know when to interject with individuals to enable them to learn themselves; being open to criticism yourself is also needed. Essentially you need to encourage and support others as well as become increasingly aware of your own emotional response to differing situations and conversations. This will enable you to build relationships, which is essential to any leader or manager within healthcare (Phillips, 2013).

To ensure you get the support needed you will need to be aware and follow your organisation's clinical supervision policy and process. Clinical supervision will form part of your learning development as well as enable you to consolidate your education as you move from student to registered practitioner.

Having a mentor and/or coach is a key area that you must think about and consider carefully. Mentors will be able to support you and share their experiences to support you, deliver care, develop yourself, and generate ideas to improve the care you and your team deliver. Coaching will support you in developing your own solutions to the challenges you face clinically, personally, or professionally and can help you work through the ethical dilemmas that you will face in your practice. Mentoring is usually a longer-term relationship as it is aimed to build confidence and support mentees to develop their skills (NHS Education for Scotland) and you may have more than one mentor. It is suggested that several mentors are beneficial to cover all aspects of your career development. Coaching tends to be a shorter-term arrangement and regularly lasts over six 1- to 2-hour sessions (NHS Education for Scotland) and may just cover a number of sessions; this will enable focus to be developed and building of a contract of outcomes that can be expected during the development sessions. Building these networks is also an essential development tool for leaders to use. Being able to call on these networks when you are unsure of actions needed in particular situations could be beneficial to you and others as you go through your career.

As Registered Nurses it is easy to become overwhelmed by the emotional impact of the care we deliver; the situations we work in and face regularly will have an effect on you personally, and being able to openly discuss these with a trusted individual to support your decision making or managing an ethical situation will help to develop your skills as a registered practitioner and will work in conjunction with your own personal reflections.

Challenging leaders or systems

Knowing when and how to celebrate good practice is equally as important as knowing when and how to challenge poor practice. In every team or service, there will be examples of good practice alongside any examples of less-than-optimal practices. However, if leadership only focuses on the negative side of things and never celebrates what a team does well, it can quickly lead to a plummeting of team morale. While identifying both positive and negative examples of practice, it is vital that you avoid falling into the trap of 'this is how we do this here' – this is how habits of poor practice manifest in areas, and they can be extremely difficult to change once ingrained. These practices become 'norms' and there are positive and negative examples of this.

Central to any change of behaviours and norms is communication. Simply criticising a poor example of practice is not going to make the positive changes that you are aiming for. This is where it is important that we communicate our views sensitively and appropriately. There is a time and a place to raise concerns, as well as good methods of communicating them. Simply saying 'you're doing this wrong' is not appropriate. However, you can encourage and influence good practice by demonstrating best practice in your work.

NMC

THE CODE SAYS

Preserve Safety

You make sure that patient and public safety is not affected. You work within the limits of your competence, exercising your professional 'duty of candour' and raising concerns immediately whenever you come across situations that put patients or public safety at risk. You take necessary action to deal with any concerns where appropriate

This provides the opportunity for observations of practice and potentially even identifying those staff members that influence the others within the clinical area. Knowing who these influencers are, regardless of their positive or negative effects, is vital to ensuring you can plan your steps of making positive change appropriately.

CASE STUDY

Rebecca Emmins, Registered Children's Nurse

Leadership has many styles which can be utilised in different scenarios to achieve positive outcomes. Rigid leaders who fail to adopt different tactics can fail to achieve effective teamwork by losing contact with their team and the team not working potentially with the same objective. Historically, nursing students were viewed as recipients of information who were expected to act a certain way and felt unable to speak out about changes until their education was completed and they had established a place in their employment. As the nursing role developed and responsibilities became greater with the development of evidence-based practice and the power change from doctor's maids to nurses assessing and critically analysing situations, this empowers the student to participate in the planning of care. As a result, leadership in this instance is of oneself, and the responsibility to ensure the nursing students not only advocating for the patient but ensuring that the care they participate in is developing their skills and achieving their planned outcomes.

Continued

CASE STUDY—cont'd

A night shift on the wards can require Registered Nurses to care for patients with fewer of the multi-disciplinary team available. Registered Nurses must use their learned knowledge to evaluate the presentation of a patient and act accordingly. On one night shift, a 13-year-old male required an injury to his leg requiring neurovascular observations. When assigned to this patient, I carried out neurovascular observations and believed the child's toes felt warmer. It was documented in the patient notes that the surgeon was to be bleeped if there were any changes. I informed a Registered Nurse and went to bleep the surgeon, but the Registered Nurses told me not to and to continue monitoring due to it being very early morning. Knowing that the injury could lead to compartment syndrome and knowing the signs, I disobeyed the Registered Nurses and went ahead and bleeped the surgeon. They arrived shortly after and reviewed the patient. It was decided that he required surgical intervention and he was taken to theatre. In theatre they discovered he had compartment syndrome and treated it, meaning the child now had a big wound to his leg. The intervention potentially saved the child from losing his leg.

Disobeying the team's decision to not contact the surgeon took leadership of myself. Confidence to stand up and advocate for a patient with evidence of my concerns empowered me to act in the best interests of the patient. I communicated clearly my actions by documenting and informing the nurse in charge. Some of the team were unsupportive but I maintained confidence in my abilities and took leadership of the situation to achieve the best outcome for the patient. I worried about my future on this placement if I was wrong to contact the surgeon.

Perceptions of leadership

Nursing students start to be assessed from their first shift in a team, and then when conducting entry interviews welcome and discuss learning outcomes. Leadership of one's own education is required where the onus is placed on the student to speak up and communicate clearly what they need to achieve. Poor leadership at this initial stage could possibly change how the team perceives you. Some Registered Nurses maintain a hierarchical approach whereby they discount the students' voice over their own as they believe that as the student is new, all their knowledge and experience is junior; however, as nursing students are no longer stereotypical single college leavers and many enter training with a wealth of experience, nursing students are informed and can voice concerns despite what the hierarchical approach followers believe.

We can see, from RE's experience, that in order to prioritise her patient as per the Code, a core attitude within the clinical area had to be openly defied. This took a substantial amount of confidence and courage on her part. It is not often that the situations faced by a student would be this drastic, with the potential for a patient to lose a limb. However, we can see that it is not impossible. We must consider the consequences of all our actions and choices in delivering care, and RE demonstrated here that putting the patient first and trusting your instincts when assessing a patient is key to ensuring safe, effective care is always delivered. Always document your discussions with staff members and your rationale for your decisions. It is the documentation that will demonstrate your capabilities should your decision making ever be questioned, which can happen months after the event. We must make challenging decisions every single day, and therefore it can be extremely difficult, if not nigh-on impossible, to remember the entire context of a particular case.

CONCLUSION

Leadership within and across nursing is a skill that nursing students need to develop using the areas identified in this chapter, as well as bring their own life skills and skills developed in other roles prior to the start of their own nursing career. It is essential that students develop these skills by accessing their mentors to discuss their development skills in clinical practice and also their academic leaders within their educational institution.

There are leaders accross nursing and healthcare, working with these people, observing how they use their skills and reflecting on what the nursing student has seen as well as thinking of the impact the leader and also the student has on other people is key to enhancing the nursing profession and ensuring quality care is influenced at all levels.

Now, that you have finished this chapter. Make some notes on what you have learned.

_____

_____

_____

_____

_____

_____

_____

_____

_____

_____

_____

_____

_____

_____

_____

REFERENCES

https://assets.publishing.service.gov.uk/government/uploads/system/uploads/attachment_data/file/279124/0947.pdf

https://assets.publishing.service.gov.uk/government/uploads/system/uploads/attachment_data/file/408480/47487_MBI_Accessible_v0.1.pdf

https://www.kingsfund.org.uk/publications/what-is-compassionate-leadership

Bradford District Care NHS Foundation Trust. (2016). *Race: Evidence of Health Inequalities Affecting Black and Minority Ethnic People*. Retrieved from Bradford District Care NHS Foundation Trust: https://www.bdct.nhs.uk/wp-content/uploads/2016/12/Race.pdf

Faculty of Medical Leadership and Management. (2015). *Leadership and Leadership Development in Health Care: The Evidence Base.* Retrieved from The King's Fund: https://www.kingsfund.org.uk/sites/default/files/field/field_publication_file/leadership-leadership-development-health-care-feb-2015.pdf

Linton M, Koonmen J. Self-care as an ethical obligation for nurses. *Nurs Ethics.* 2020 Jul 28:969733020940371. doi:10.1177/0969733020940371. Epub ahead of print.

Mlambo M, Silén C, McGrath C. Lifelong learning and nurses' continuing professional development, a metasynthesis of the literature. *BMC Nurs.* 2021 Apr 14;20(1):62. doi:10.1186/s12912-021-00579-2.

NHS England. (2017). *Improving Through Inclusion: Supporting Staff Networks for Black and Minority Ethnic Staff in the NHS.* Retrieved from NHS England: https://www.england.nhs.uk/wp-content/uploads/2017/08/inclusion-report-aug-2017.pdf

NHS Leadership Academy. (2013). *Healthcare Leadership Model.* Retrieved from NHS Leadership Academy: https://www.leadershipacademy.nhs.uk/resources/healthcare-leadership-model/

Nursing and Midwifery Council. (2018). *The Code.* Retrieved from Nursing and Midwifery Council: https://www.nmc.org.uk/globalassets/sitedocuments/nmc-publications/nmc-code.pdf

Patel KM, Metersky K. Reflective practice in nursing: A concept analysis. *Int J Nurs Knowl.* 2022 Jul;33(3):180-187. doi:10.1111/2047-3095.12350. Epub 2021 Oct 9.

Pinder, R. J., Ferguson, J., & Møller, H. (2016). Minority ethnicity patient satisfaction and experience: Results of the National Cancer Patient Experience Survey in England. *British Medical Journal (Open Access).* doi:10.1136/bmjopen-2016-011938

Royal College of Nursing. (2022). *Clinical Governance: Leadership.* Retrieved from Royal College of Nursing: https://www.rcn.org.uk/clinical-topics/clinical-governance/leadership

Scully NJ. Leadership in nursing: The importance of recognising inherent values and attributes to secure a positive future for the profession. *Collegian.* 2015;22(4):439-44. doi:10.1016/j.colegn.2014.09.004.

Tomey, A. M. (2008). Nursing leadership and management effects work environments. *Journal of Nursing Management, 17*(1), 15–25. doi: 10.1111/j.1365-2834.2008.00963.x

Valiga TM. Leaders, managers, and followers: Working in harmony. *Nursing.* 2019 Jan;49(1):45-48. doi:10.1097/01.NURSE.0000549723.07316.0b.

Nursing and Midwifery Council Social Media Guidance. (2019). https://www.nmc.org.uk/standards/guidance/social-media-guidance/read-social-media-guidance-online/

NHS Education for Scotland Coaching and mentoring in health and care | Turas | Learn (nhs.scot)

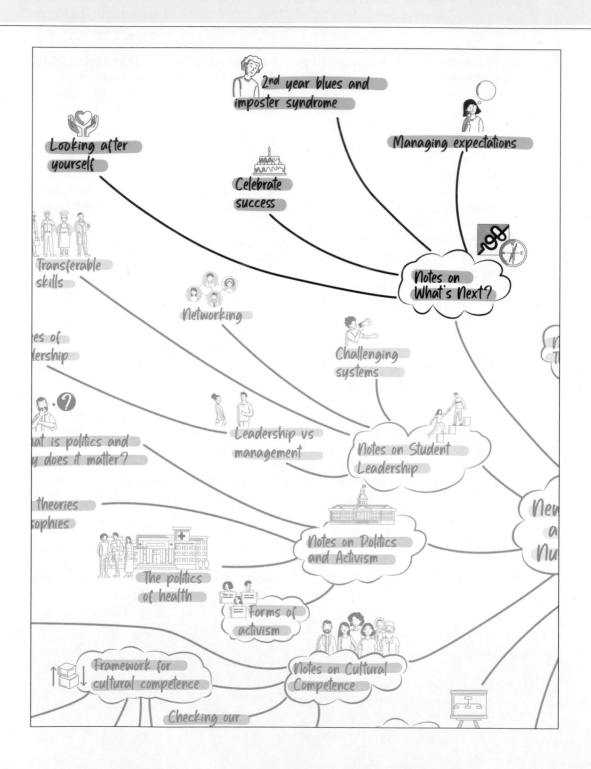

NOTES ON WHAT NEXT?

Chelsea Fawcett (She/Her) ■ Elisha Woolf (She/Her)
■ Emma Hall (She/Her)

INTRODUCTION

This chapter aims to address what to expect after you have completed your first year of nursing studies. You may be feeling a mixture of emotions as you embark on the next part of your journey, but you are certainly not alone and the thoughts of other nursing students in a similar position have been included to demonstrate that. Now that you have completed the first year, you are in a good position to reflect on your experience so far and consider how you want to tackle the next year.

Managing your workload and your work-life balance will be essential as you progress, and this chapter looks at helpful ways you can do this. You may have started to compare yourself to other nursing students, and the following section aims to help you to acknowledge this and think about what you can learn from this.

There will be a brief discussion around imposter syndrome and the second-year blues, which you may or may not experience over the next year or so, but it's best to be prepared for this and have some coping strategies up your sleeve.

What's more, you may be wondering what to actually expect after your first year. You may be worried about having more responsibilities and learning new skills, and the authors of this chapter share knowledge from their own experiences of being a nursing student to guide you.

Lastly, it's a good time to briefly consider what comes after second year, so you can take the next steps hopefully feeling more prepared and confident about what is to come.

THE MIXED EMOTIONS AROUND BECOMING A SECOND-YEAR NURSING STUDENT

You may be reading this as you are about to begin your second year of nursing studies. You might be feeling a mixture of emotions during your transition from first year to second year, and that's understandable. As you have completed your first year you will already be aware that the nursing degree is very time consuming, requiring a large amount of dedication and commitment.

In a tweet asking nursing students how they felt about starting their second year of nursing studies, people expressed feeling apprehensive about the changes in academic requirements. Tweets that stood out were:

TWEET

@amymann92:

Petrified, excited, nervous but somehow part of me is ready!'

TWEET

@JoJo_RosaStN:

'I'm currently on placement and 2 weeks away from finishing placement and that's first-year completed. I'm looking forward to going on holiday before I start second year in September. I'm feeling both excited and nervous to start the next stage in my future career in nursing'

TWEET

@ChloeHHScott:

'I'm excited to finally say I'm a 2nd year student! But I am absolutely terrified. I've heard that 2nd year is one of the hardest. Even though this year I am passing with grades above 70 - I'm worried I will need to drop out due to the pressure that placement brings'

From the responses, it was clear that feelings were mixed. Feeling nervous about starting a new chapter in your journey to becoming a registered nurse is understandable. Firstly, the grades you achieve going forward will now count towards your final degree classification (depending on your place of study). Secondly, there may be some expectations that being a second-year nursing student means having more knowledge and responsibility than a first-year nursing student. Thirdly, you may have heard rumours about 'Second year blues' or that second year is the most challenging year. With all these concepts, a feeling of fear and apprehension is only natural. The important thing to remember here is that many of these pressures come from within.

FINDING A BALANCE

One of these pressures is that life can quickly become all about nursing – not just through studying and being on placement but consuming nursing and healthcare-related social media, books, and TV shows. It can sometimes feel like you are living and breathing nursing. You are going from university, to placement, and then home where you are studying, maybe spending time on social media talking about current nursing issues and networking. It's important to give yourself permission to take a break.

When things start to feel like this, it is worth starting to structure your week. Keeping lists can be helpful, perhaps keeping a diary or a weekly/monthly spreadsheet so that you can see what your commitments are. By doing this you can see where you are spending too much time working and 'nursing' and not enough down time. The image below was created to demonstrate how everything in life can overlap as a nursing student but it all forms part of your identity.

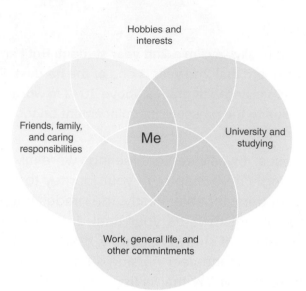

Hobbies and
interests

Friends, family,
and caring
responsibilities

Me

University and
studying

Work, general life, and
other commintments

With all of this going on it's okay to recognise that it can all be a bit much sometimes. This could look like seeing other people's achievements when you don't feel like you are doing as well as everyone else. You may find yourself comparing yourself to others too much. This is a sign to turn it off for a while so that you can reconnect with the things that matter the most to you. Take the time to step away completely so that you can breathe and get headspace; there is no harm in taking time away so that you can achieve a healthier work-life balance.

Maybe you have a part-time job in healthcare, and conversations ultimately revolve around nursing. As a result, we can start to lose sight of who we are outside of being a nursing student. You still have a way to go before becoming a registered nurse, so it's important to take the time now to look after yourself so that you can be there for others. When you finish university and register as a nurse, the habits you formed whilst a student can help you to form a better work-life balance for when you do become a registered nurse.

It can be easy to quickly become overwhelmed and this affects your life in and out of university. You may have found that you don't have time for your hobbies or other commitments. Friendships, relationships, and your social life may be suffering. Perhaps you can't work many shifts at your paid job, or you feel guilty as you don't have as much time to spend with your children or take your dog for a walk. Or, whenever you are doing something that's not university related, you end up thinking about it or feeling guilty that you aren't doing university work!

If you've felt this way or if you do feel this way in the future, especially moving into your second year, what can be done to manage this? How do we maintain both our physical and mental health needs to carry out our future professional role as nurses, as set out by the Code (NMC, 2018)?

NMC

THE CODE SAYS

20.9 'maintain the level of health you need to carry out your professional role'

Ultimately, managing your time effectively will be particularly advantageous in retaining your identity and sense of self outside of being a nursing student. This will allow you to keep and build on your interests outside of nursing, so your life does not revolve around healthcare and studying. Here are a few suggestions:

TIP

- If you need to work part-time, consider a job that is outside of healthcare – in a supermarket or bartending, for example. Or, consider bank work, where you can do as many or few shifts as you have time for.

TIP

- Utilise self-directed study time allocated to you by university and avoid having to do that work in your own time.

TIP

- Try putting certain 'rules' in place to help keep free time that's not university related! For example – no university work to be done after 7 pm, or work on assignments either on Saturday OR Sunday but not both.

TIP

- Schedule – Use a diary/planner. Not just to record lectures, shifts, and dates to see friends and family, but schedule 'me time' for hobbies, a bath, a run, or time to read a book. Not everyone likes a schedule but give it a try – even just to loosely plan your week out.

TIP

- Try small group study with others on your course. You can all work on getting work done together but also socialise!

TIP

- Be honest with friends and family about your workload, and what you're finding tough. Whilst they may not exactly understand, they can offer advice and a different perspective.

Balancing workload is an important part of managing the overlapping demands mentioned above. When the workload increases in the second year of being a nursing student, it can become challenging to spend time doing things that are not nursing related. You might find that you are '*shoulding*' yourself. This might look like thoughts such as, 'I *should* be doing more at university, I *should* help with that open day, I *should* volunteer for that project, I *should* be joining societies'.

Although you may enjoy taking on extra-curricular activities within nursing, and it can certainly be of benefit to your career, it can be easy to take on too much and potentially leave you ending up feeling burnt out and overwhelmed with the world of healthcare. It can also add an obligation to something which was supposed to be a fun activity or interesting learning opportunity. It could leave you feeling resentful or put unnecessary pressure on something you believe you are *supposed to be doing*.

Remember, you are not expected to take on any extra-curricular activities at university. But if you find yourself faced with one or several opportunities and would like to take one or two on, consider each one and how it can benefit you and work within your lifestyle. Think about:

- Which will be of most benefit to my learning/career?
- Which will be the most enjoyable?
- Are any of these opportunities flexible with my time?
- Do I really want to do this, or do I feel obligated to give my time?
- Will any of these opportunities be available to access later?

THIS IS YOUR UNIQUE JOURNEY

You may find yourself comparing yourself to others; your academic work and grades, your performance on placement, opportunities, and awards that never seem to come your way. Or you may have peers that seem to be breezing through the course, whereas you feel it has been more of a struggle.

In a conversation with a nursing student, Ellie stated,

> *'I once heard a quote that you should never measure yourself using someone else's ruler. I realised this is what I had been doing and it was making me miserable'.*

These thoughts and feelings – although often common – can have a negative impact on your motivation, mental health, and even friendships if you find yourself constantly comparing your achievements and progress to others. This might look like:

- Poor motivation – avoiding doing assignments or revision with the fear of failing.
- Low self-esteem.
- Negative self-talk.
- Difficulty with friendships if you become jealous or resentful of others' 'ease' to complete assignments/placement.
- Setting difficult or unattainable goals and then being hard on yourself if you don't meet them.

- Taking on extra-curricular work or commitments to prove to yourself that you are capable, but then having an even bigger workload and added pressure.

There are several ways you can try to combat this, and different things will work for different people. Firstly, acknowledge that these feelings are completely natural, but the key is to not let these feelings take control of your thoughts and your actions. Most people on your course will be feeling the same way; they may just be good at hiding it! Remind yourself that no one can be the best or be good at everything, and it is okay not to be perfect. Everyone has their own strengths, achievements, and areas for growth. Don't compare yourself and your 'behind the scenes' to other people's highlight reel.

You could start by accepting any past errors or mistakes – you have learned from these. If there are areas you feel you genuinely need to work on, acknowledge these and plan or write a goal based on feedback you have received. Ensure that you are setting these goals for your own self-development rather than in comparison to others. Using SMART goal-setting (specific, measurable, achievable, relevant, and time-bound) (Doran, 1981) is a great way to make a goal attainable within a set timeframe.

CASE STUDY

Amanda had a meeting with her practice assessor and identified that she did not feel confident about administering intramuscular injections. Together they set the following goal: arrange to spend a day with a nurse at the depot clinic before the mid-point review. To prepare for this, read around the theory and guidelines, observe some injections taking place, and when ready administer at least three intramuscular injections to patients under supervision. Amanda and her assessor both agreed that this specified the goal, was measurable by the number of injections to administer, was achievable because there would be plenty of opportunities to administer injections, was relevant to Amanda's end-of-placement assessment, and was time-bound as there was a realistic deadline.

Rather than setting one large goal, break it down into smaller more manageable goals — this will give you a sense of achievement as you tick each one off the list. If you have peers that have already achieved this task, maybe they can help you meet your goal?

It can be easy to centre your attention on what you haven't done, what others have achieved, or how far behind you perceive yourself to be. It is important to remember how far you have come and what you have achieved. This is your unique journey.

Here is just one summary of a unique journey:

TWEET

(@PhoebeJayeMiles)

Phoebe started her newly registered nurse journey in critical care before moving to research nursing and studying for a Master's degree part-time and then moved to China to do a PhD.

What is important to acknowledge here is that your nursing journey will look different to others'. There is no such thing as a typical nursing journey. Many nursing students interrupt their studies, need to re-sit placements or exams, or start off in one field of nursing before moving to another field entirely.

You will all meet targets at different times, achieve different successes, and have varying struggles. You may feel that you are lacking knowledge or skills in a certain area, and your peers on the course may be able to help you with this, and vice versa. You will learn with and from each other — and this will continue throughout your nursing career as you evolve and develop as a nurse in an ever-changing profession.

Take a moment to reflect on your strengths and achievements so far; try to think of three things you feel confident at performing or doing within your nursing degree or in your personal life.

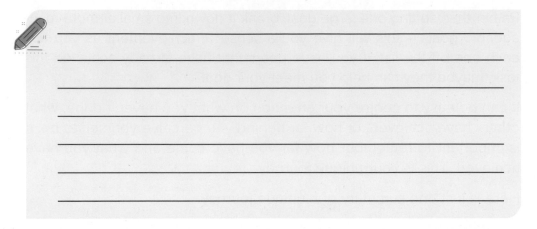

Celebrate others' successes as well as your own. If you have received a lower grade than you had hoped for, have not known the answer to something in class, or have struggled with a placement, sometimes it can feel difficult to be happy for others. This doesn't make you selfish or a bad person, but it can lead to feelings of resentment towards others or yourself. Aim to celebrate that success as if it was your own – the happiness and positivity you feel from doing this can lead to greater optimism and motivation for yourself to reach that same goal!

Additionally, do your best not to let fear or comparison guide your choices and decisions. Don't take on a project or extra-curricular activities just because you see your peers doing this. Think your idea for an assignment seems too easy or plain compared to someone else's? Stick to what you want to do – if you're within the guidelines of the assignment, it is much easier to write about a subject you are passionate about! You want to be able to look back on your time studying your degree with overall fondness and pride, not with regret over what you 'should' have done (remember 'shoulding').

These feelings may reflect how you will feel in the future when you embark on your career. As both a nursing student and registered nurse, you are expected to act under the Code of Conduct.

NMC | THE CODE SAYS

To practice effectively, nurses are encouraged to 'gather and reflect on feedback from various sources, using it to improve your practice and performance'

One area you can prepare for is the change in what is expected of you in your academic writing and your practice in your second year. For example, some of you may be writing at level five instead of level four, and you will be expected to be more critical in your writing (Carmichael, 2019).

Take a moment to reflect on what you think is expected of you as a second-year nursing student. This can be a reflection on your expectations, the perceived expectations of others, or what you have heard from others. Try to be as honest as you can. Once you have exhausted your list, speak to other nursing students about the list – you may find that others are feeling the same way.

_____

_____

_____

_____

_____

_____

_____

Next, arrange a meeting with your academic supervisor or your practice assessor and discuss your list in more detail. It may be that some of your expectations are realistic, and you can formulate a plan together.

On the other hand, it may be that your expectations are unrealistic (remember SMART goals) and having a frank conversation about this may remove some of the pressure you may be feeling. By doing this, you are setting yourself up to be a reflective practitioner who is mindful of their performance and strives for continuous self-development to improve the patient experience.

The above section talked about comparing yourself to others and dealing with setbacks. On the contrary, you may be feeling like you haven't learned anything in your first year, or even that you don't know enough to be a second-year nursing student. Now is the time to pause, reflect, and plan.

Try to reflect on the past year and think back to the introduction chapter of this book, where you were asked to set your goals and objectives. You may need to refer to your journal, class notes, or other documentation to jog your memory.

Choose three things you have learned in the past year and write them down. If you can think of more, that's brilliant too!

After doing this, hopefully, you will surprise yourself and realise how far you have come already.

IMPOSTER SYNDROME

In addition to the pressure you may be feeling about embarking on your second year, you may be familiar with the phenomenon of imposter syndrome. The term 'imposter syndrome' originates from the 1970s and is used to describe a feeling of 'believing that they are really not bright and have fooled anyone who thinks otherwise' (Clance and Imes, 1978). Despite all your achievements, you are left feeling like an imposter and this is a feeling that can be difficult to shake (Day-Calder, 2017). As a nursing student this can hinder your ability to focus, along with impacting your wellbeing. This can be difficult to overcome, both as a nursing student and as a newly registered nurse.

In a discussion with newly registered nurse Emily, she said, 'I found it really difficult being a NQN. There is always that little voice telling me "you're not cut out for this", or "you're not like everyone else here". I found it really helpful to talk to someone who I trusted at work to let them know how I was feeling and seek their advice' (personal communication).

So how do you overcome this? Truth be told, it's not easy to start with, but it can get easier. Think about whether your thoughts are a fact or opinion. For example, if you think you are not good enough, what is the evidence for and against this? Is there evidence that this is a fact, and if so, what can you do to change this? It is likely, however, that this is your own opinion, so think about the evidence that demonstrates you *are* good enough – your grades, positive feedback from assessors and patients, and things you have learned that you never knew before becoming a nursing student. Remember to speak with your academic and practice assessors if you are struggling with thoughts like this so that you can work together to build your confidence.

Remember, you are not alone in feeling like this and over time you will come to recognise how much you have achieved and that you have earned your place. The people assessing you are responsible for ensuring you are suitable to become a registered nurse, and they would not allow you to continue if they thought otherwise. You succeeded in getting a place on the course, and you have passed your assignments and placements so far to be able to start your second year, so you must be doing something right! Believe in yourself like others believe in you.

SECOND-YEAR BLUES

As a nursing student, you may have heard of second-year blues before. In a recent blog post, a nursing student described second-year blues as a feeling of 'limbo' and a 'drop in momentum' after putting so much energy into the first year (The Pint-Sized Student Nurse, 2019). Another nursing student described feeling so low in their second year that they needed to seek help from their GP (Toni, 2019).

'As a first-year nursing student, I found the workload easy to manage and I thought the degree was going to be a walk in the park. I'd heard about second-year blues but I thought to myself, that won't be me. As second year began, I started to find the work more challenging, and began feeling anxious about the standard of my work. Then the pandemic hit, and everything became much more difficult to manage. I felt anxious that without face-to-face lectures, I would fail my assignments. The pandemic was unexpected, but I think I would have struggled anyway. In the end, I sought support from my university's student services department and my GP, and was able to stay on track with my course. The point is, three years is a long time, and a nursing degree is very challenging. I wish that I'd felt more prepared, not for second-year blues, but for any kind of blues'.

–Chelsea Fawcett, Registered Nurse

Helping yourself through a difficult time

There is no certainty that every nursing student will experience this phenomenon; however, being a nursing student is challenging. It is therefore essential to prepare ways to look after your mental health throughout your entire degree. As you are just about to embark on your second year, why not take some time now to do this?

You could create a safety plan, which is an evidence-based method of preparing for a mental health crisis (Staying Safe, 2022). Start by making a list of things you would want yourself to know if you were struggling, or perhaps some positive feedback you have received. Include specific people you could contact such as friends, family members, student support services, or mental health helplines.

Write down ways you can distract yourself and things that you usually find calming or soothing.

_____

_____

_____

_____

_____

_____

Having this written down in preparation for a time when you might be struggling could really help you to work through that specific moment so that you are able to come up with a plan of how to solve your problem. A helpful website for creating your own safety plan is stayingsafe.net.

Alternatively, you could create a self-soothe box filled with sensory things that can help you to keep calm in a crisis (Young Minds, 2019). For example, find a nice box and add items like scented candles, sour sweets, fidget toys, and your favourite book or movie. You can be as creative as you like with items that help you to feel calm and grounded. Put the box somewhere safe and when you start to feel overwhelmed you can get the box out.

What might you put into your box?

_____

_____

_____

_____

_____

_____

WHAT YOU MIGHT EXPECT FROM YOURSELF AS A SECOND-YEAR NURSING STUDENT

Turning now to expectations on nursing students in second year, you may feel that there is an added expectation or responsibility onto your skills and capabilities. You've made it through your first year, and you might feel that you're not a 'beginner' anymore and when you get out into placement or back into the classroom there is going to be more expected of you. You may well be doubting your abilities and feel more pressure is being put on you or that voice in your head is telling you, 'I can't do this!'. You certainly aren't alone; everyone feels like this from time to time. So how can you manage these expectations and extra responsibilities?

Here is a little bit of theory to put this into perspective:

Dr Patricia Benner developed the 'Stages of Clinical Competence' (Benner and Benner, 2001). There are five stages of potential assessment; these are Stage 1: Novice, Stage 2: Advanced Beginner, Stage 3: Competent, Stage 4: Proficient, and Stage 5: Expert. One main theme among nursing students is self-doubt and the lack of ability to assess themselves accordingly (Aller, 2021).

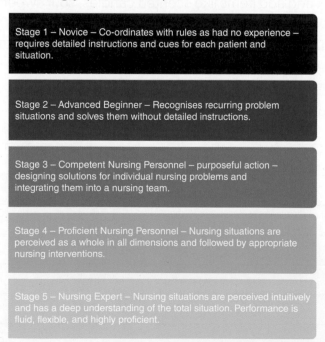

Stage 1 – Novice – Co-ordinates with rules as had no experience – requires detailed instructions and cues for each patient and situation.

Stage 2 – Advanced Beginner – Recognises recurring problem situations and solves them without detailed instructions.

Stage 3 – Competent Nursing Personnel – purposeful action – designing solutions for individual nursing problems and integrating them into a nursing team.

Stage 4 – Proficient Nursing Personnel – Nursing situations are perceived as a whole in all dimensions and followed by appropriate nursing interventions.

Stage 5 – Nursing Expert – Nursing situations are perceived intuitively and has a deep understanding of the total situation. Performance is fluid, flexible, and highly proficient.

Figure 10.1   Benner's Stages of Clinical Competence.

The 'Stages of Clinical Competence' is a useful tool to help with this when looking at self-assessment. This can be used at any time with any aspect of your development. For example, looking at nursing students, generally they would be placed in Stage 1: Novice (Figure 10.1). A nursing student in their first years of clinical education would have limited foresight or ability to predict what might happen in each situation due to their limited nursing experience.

This tool can be used generally, and it can also be used for more specific instances such as learning a new skill informally or formally. Self-assessment and self-feedback are an important part of a nursing student's learning and development and your ability to assess where you are in terms of your confidence. Informal self-assessment can be enough to help you see things in perspective so that you can move on and grow.

That's enough theory for now (Fig 10.1). Everyone is guilty of putting high expectations on themselves from time to time. Despite the expectations we put on ourselves, no one is perfect. You are only human. Manage your own expectations, and take the time to self-reflect on your competence – you are not going to know everything there is to know about a particular subject and you can forgive yourself for that. Every moment and experience is a learning opportunity. Take notes, reflect on how you feel, and set small goals to improve or approach it differently next time.

EXTRA RESPONSIBILITIES

As you transition to second year you may be asked to do more on clinical placement and in your academic work. However, it is important to remember that you will only ever be expected to work within your competency, which varies from person to person. It is important to talk to your practice assessor about your current levels of confidence and competence so that they can work with you effectively. Remind yourself of your reflections from earlier on how far you have come, your level of confidence, and what you would like to work on.

Identify your level of confidence. This might seem like a strange statement, but as a nursing student you will progress and there will come a time when you start to question your abilities and your confidence. You may find you are starting to do a lot more and take more responsibility under minimal supervision and guidance. If you start to question your confidence this is a good time to look back on how far you've come and read the positive feedback you've received in the past. This can give you the boost you need to keep moving forward.

Your academic work may be more in depth. You'll be reading wider and delving deeper into subjects. Your university or college will talk about critical analysis, databases, Boolean phrases, and qualitative research and at placement you might be starting to hear them ask you if you want to take a team of patients, complete the medications round, or do some paperwork on your own with some supervision but not as much as you are used to. What's more, the skills you develop in second year may be different to those of other nursing students, as everyone's journey is different (different placement experiences and different assessment topics, for example). Seems like a lot, right?

 TIP

Tips to get you started

Try to take things one day at a time if things are getting too much. Remember, you are still a student, and you are there to have supportive, constructive, protected learning. Whose expectation are you aiming to fulfil? Is it the expectation of the university/placement? Or is it the expectation you have put on yourself? If it is the latter, are you putting too much pressure on yourself?

 TIP

Tips to get you started

Try and keep an open mind about the given situation. Are you dwelling on the negatives? 'This is too hard', 'I can't do this' – these sorts of negative thought trails can lead to spiralling, when really by keeping a more open mind you can aim to change how you think to a more positive train of thoughts. Turn those negative statements into more positive ones; for example: 'This is hard but what small thing can I achieve today?'.

If you have really high expectations of yourself, you'll burn out too quickly. It can be helpful to look at each shift or day with a different perspective and approach. If you are struggling it can be helpful to assess each day accordingly, focusing on the positives however small they may seem. Everyone learns at a different pace and in a different way. You are a student, and you are learning. It is perfectly acceptable to say, 'please could you show me again' or 'can we just go over this again.' You will be surprised how many people need to do things multiple times before something sinks in or your learning consolidates enough for it all to click together.

You may or may not have heard about clinical supervision as a nursing student but it's worth taking the time to consider early in your career. For those of you who have never heard about clinical supervision, it's a time for you to reflect with another or in a group on your practice (Bond and Holland, 1998). It is not about counselling or managerial supervision but a time to think about your practice and how you can develop yourself for future practice.

For example, you might use a clinical supervision session to reflect on a challenging conversation you had with a patient. You could explore why you felt it was challenging and you may find that others can share their knowledge and wisdom with you. You may feel unsure about how to develop your skills in this area and your clinical supervisor may be able to signpost you to the right place.

When you are next on a placement, ask about clinical supervision and see if you can access it during your time there as a nursing student. Ask the nursing staff if they have had clinical supervision and what they find helpful/unhelpful. Reflect on any barriers to clinical supervision in practice and how you might overcome these as a registered nurse to ensure you get protected time for this valuable reflective practice.

_____

_____

_____

_____

_____

_____

THINKING A LITTLE FURTHER AHEAD

We've spent some time talking about what to expect in your second year. As a first-year nursing student this is the next step, so why look any further ahead? Well, thinking ahead to third year can be beneficial. You don't need to think about it too much, but it is helpful to at least acknowledge it and understand where your studies are headed. Depending on your course you may be expected to write a dissertation or a service improvement project. It is worth bearing this in mind when you are working on your current assignments.

For example, you may need to be able to run a database search to find literature for your project. The last thing you want to be doing when taking on such a huge piece of work is learning some of the basics, when you could be learning them in your second year. If database searches sound daunting, they don't have to be.

Take the time to learn how to search for literature further than your reading list, and add your notes on what you find

_____

_____

_____

_____

_____

_____

_____

CASE STUDY

Sarah wanted to learn about a particular disease. This was a perfect opportunity to try a literature search using a database, to find the most relevant and up-to-date information on her chosen topic. She booked an appointment with the subject librarian to learn more about how to run an effective database search and get the most out of the library. After the appointment, Sarah felt more confident about database searches and this made completing future assignments less daunting. These skills not only helped with completing assignments but were carried forward when she was expected to give a presentation for a job interview later in her career, and when she wanted to learn more about specific nursing interventions in her new job.

If you really want to look ahead, you will find this skill valuable as a registered nurse when updating your knowledge and participating in service improvements. Keeping your knowledge and skills up to date with evidence-based information is an essential part of the NMC *Code*.

NMC

THE CODE SAYS

6.2 maintain the knowledge and skills you need for safe and effective practice

Literature searching is only one skill you may need to be well versed in by third year, but there will be other skills too.

Think about what these skills might be and speak with your academic supervisor to start working towards those skills at an earlier stage. Then, practise the skills you've learned for your next assignment or your next placement. Your future self will thank you.

_____

_____

_____

_____

_____

_____

_____

Top tips for first-year nursing students thinking ahead

TIP

'Schedule in time off if you find things are getting too much. You can't pour from an empty cup. Be mindful of making time for mindfulness to recharge with the things you love to do and the people you love to be around'.

TWEET

@NQN_ Jenniee

'Take time for yourself & breathe. It might be the longest 3 or 4 years of your life, but its only 3 or 4 years!'.

TWEET

@Chelsea14878

'You'll never know everything and that's ok!'.

TWEET

@HayleyL_Pollock

'Keep a journal of things you do well/stories that make you smile. It helps to reflect on the bad days'.

'Be kind to yourself and remember this is your journey and no-one else's'.

—Emma Hall, Registered Nurse

'Your grades should not define you. That does not mean you shouldn't try your hardest and be the best you can be, but what it does mean is you need to recognise when you are pushing yourself too far. When you receive your grade, will you be proud of yourself, or will you be too exhausted to appreciate your hard work? Do your best but look after yourself in the process. Eat well, drink water, exercise, socialise and do what's important to you, but most of all be kind to yourself. You can't do better than your best'.

– Chelsea Fawcett, Registered Nurse

CONCLUSION

Second year is going to be challenging, but it is achievable. Hopefully the subjects talked about in this section can be a helpful hint to pointing you in a new direction or casting a different perspective on a given situation to help you tackle the future. Always remember to be kind to yourself; you are valued at university, and you are valued at placement. Completing your course is going to be tough but the nurses out there are living proof that it can be done, as are the cohort in front of you.

Be patient with yourself and those around you. You are learning all the time, so if you can take time to lean on others and let others lean on you in return for their time of need. Ask for help when you need it. You may have sleepless nights and longer days than you have ever imagined, but you'll get through second year and over that peak before you know it and then it's all downhill to the finish line. Hopefully some of the tips and strategies shared in this chapter can help you to feel more confident about starting your second year of nursing studies and may help you as your progress even further. By taking the time now to prepare for the year ahead, you've done one of the hardest parts.

Now, that you have finished this chapter. Make some notes on what you have learned.

_____

_____

_____

_____

_____

_____

_____

_____

_____

_____

_____

_____

_____

_____

_____

_____

_____

_____

_____

_____

REFERENCES

https://www.youngminds.org.uk/young-person/blog/how-to-make-a-self-soothe-box/

Aller, L. (2021). 'A Contemporary Model for Undergraduate Nursing Education: A Grounded Theory Study', *Nurse Educator,* vol. 46/no. 4, pp. 250–254.

Benner, P. (2001). *From Novice to Expert: Excellence and Power in Clinical Nursing Practice*, Anonymous Translator (Prentice Hall).

Carmichael, C. (2019). *Second year preparation: What do you need?* [Online]. Available at: https://www.bing.com/videos/search?q=preparing+for+2nd+year+claire+carmichael&&view=detail&mid=5BDEF6BCB48EDDE7953C5BDEF6BCB48EDDE7953C&&FORM=VRDGAR&ru=%2Fvideos%2Fsearch%3Fq%3Dpreparing%2Bfor%2B2nd%2Byear%2Bclaire%2Bcarmichael%26FORM%3DHDRSC3. Accessed 4 October 2021.

Clance, P. R., & Imes, S. A. (1978). The imposter phenomenon in high achieving women: Dynamics and therapeutic intervention. Psychotherapy: Theory, Research & Practice, 15(3), 241–247. https://doi.org/10.1037/h0086006

Day-Calder, M. (2017). The perils of imposter syndrome. *Nursing Standard.* Available at: https://rcni.com/nursing-standard/students/advice-and-development/perils-of-imposter-syndrome-88241. Accessed 11 July 2022.

Doran, G. (1981). *There's a S.M.A.R.T. way to write management goals and objectives.* Available at: https://community.mis.temple.edu/mis0855002fall2015/files/2015/10/S.M.A.R.T-Way-Management-Review.pdf. Accessed 22 July 2022.

Nursing and Midwifery Council (NMC) (2018). *The code: Professional standards of practice and behaviour for nurses, midwives, and nursing associates.* London: Nursing and Midwifery Council.

Skills of clinical supervision for nurses: A practical guide for supervisees, clinical supervisors and managers (Supervision in Context)

Staying Safe (2022). *Staying safe from suicidal thoughts.* Available at: stayingsafe.net. Accessed 22 July 2022.

The Pint-Sized Student Nurse. (2019). *Second year blues. a myth or reality?* [Online]. Available at: https://thepintsizedstudentnurse.home.blog/2019/09/07/second-year-blues-a-myth-or-reality/. Accessed 4 October 2021.

Toni. (2019). *Getting through the second-year blues.* [Online]. Available at: https://www.rcn.org.uk/magazines/students/2019/getting-through-the-second-year-blues.   Accessed 4 October 2021.